T0215366

Motherhood, Spirituality and Culture

Motherhood, Spirituality and Culture explores spiritual skills that may assist women in changes, challenges and transformations undergone through the transition to motherhood. This study comprises rich, qualitative data gathered from interviews with 11 mothers. Results are analysed by constructing seven unique maternal narratives that elucidate and give voice to the mothers in their transition by in depth exploration of six themes emerging from the analysis. Overall discussion ranges across such realities as:

- desires, expectations and illusions for mothering;
- birth and spiritual embodied experiences of mothering;
- instinctual knowing; identity and crisis, and connections of motherhood;
- changes and transformations undergone through motherhood.

This study presents a unique framework for qualitative studies of spirituality within motherhood research; by weaving together transpersonal psychology, humanistic psychology, spiritual intelligence and the spiritual maternal literature. This book will appeal to all women who have transitioned to motherhood. It will also be of assistance to professionals who wish to approach any aspect of maternity care and support from a transpersonal perspective. It will also provide unique insights for academics and postgraduate students in the fields of anthropology, psychology, psychotherapy and feminism studies.

Noelia Molina, PhD is a psychotherapist, lecturer and researcher. She has been engaged in spirituality studies, workshops and teaching for more than a decade. Her PhD investigated the transition to motherhood as spiritual process. Currently she teaches several modules on the MA in Applied Spirituality accredited by Waterford Institute of Technology and hosted by the Spirituality Institute for Research and Education (SpIRE) in Dublin. She also serves on the leadership team of the programme and on the advisory board of SpIRE.

Routledge Research in Nursing and Midwifery

www.routledge.com/Routledge-Research-in-Nursing/book-series/RRIN

Motherhood, Spirituality and Culture

Noelia Molina

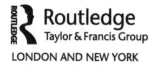
Routledge
Taylor & Francis Group

LONDON AND NEW YORK

First published 2019 by Routledge

2 Park Square, Milton Park, Abingdon, Oxon OX14 4RN

605 Third Avenue, New York, NY 10017

Routledge is an imprint of the Taylor & Francis Group, an informa business

First issued in paperback 2021

British Library Cataloguing-in-Publication Data
A catalogue record for this book is available from the British Library

Library of Congress Cataloging-in-Publication Data
Names: Molina, Noelia, author.
Title: Motherhood, spirituality and culture / Noelia Molina.
Other titles: Routledge research in nursing and midwifery.
Description: Abingdon, Oxon ; New York, NY : Routledge, 2019. | Series: Routledge research in nursing and midwifery | Includes bibliographical references and index.
Identifiers: LCCN 2018053726 | ISBN 9781138601376 (hardback) | ISBN 9780429470127 (e-book)
Subjects: LCSH: Mothers–Psychology. | Motherhood. | Spirituality. | MESH: Mothers–psychology | Spirituality | Maternal Behavior–psychology | Pregnancy–psychology
Classification: LCC HQ759.M8415 2019 | NLM HQ 759 | DDC 155.6/463–dc23
LC record available at https://lccn.loc.gov/2018053726

ISBN: 978-1-138-60137-6 (hbk)
ISBN: 978-1-03-217835-6 (pbk)
DOI: 10.4324/9780429470127

Typeset in Times New Roman
by Wearset Ltd, Boldon, Tyne and Wear

.

I wrote this book for the following people, and to them I would like to dedicate the finished product:

My two grandmothers, Ana Marchena R.I.P. and Ana Ranjel R.I.P., both children of the Spanish Civil War, who mothered the only way they could and knew.

My mother, Consuelo Palacios, who became a mother at 17 years old.

My children, Ana and Oisin. I could not have written this book if you both were not here. You were the inspiration and the source. You are both the future.

Contents

PART IV
Motherhood and spiritual care 165

Illustrations

Figure

Tables

Acknowledgements

I am grateful to many, who in different ways have helped me in the completion of my study and the writing of this book.

First, to my mother who always encouraged me since I was a child and praised all my school work while I was growing up. Her reassurance made me trust my own abilities and intellect.

To my teachers and mentors through the years, in particular, Ann Cahill R.I.P., who guided me through an important period of my life with patience, compassion and care.

To all the inspirational teachers whom I encountered in my spirituality studies in Milltown Institute of Theology and Philosophy, with a special mention of Dr Michael O'Sullivan, who was the first person in whom I confided my desire to do a PhD and who put me in contact with Dr Bernadette Flanagan.

To the students I encountered while lecturing and supervising in the MA in Applied Spirituality. They challenged my thinking and I learnt so much from them and their life experiences.

To the mothers I have counselled during these years through the maternal transition. They will never know how much strength I got from them and their stories.

To my friends, Caitriona and Nicola, for listening, and for engaging in maternal conversations with me. They reassured me constantly that I needed to do this research.

To my mother-in-law, Kantha, whose help was invaluable to me. She helped me so much with the care of my children through the process.

I want to make special mention of the women I interviewed. They were so generous, open and flexible with me and I feel privileged to have been the recipient of their maternal stories.

In those long evenings, when the kids had gone to sleep, and I settled to continuing writing, I also want to acknowledge the warm presence of my puppy Frodo, R.I.P., who lay beside me, sleeping soundly with that mysterious and strange connection that human beings have with animals.

I managed to finish my research and this book with the help of two main people who were my fully support and empowerment.

Dr Bernadette Flanagan, whose commitment, integrity and intellect inspired me to keep going. She has an internal strength and an ability to empower other women. I am indebted to her for helping me to find that internal power in myself.

My husband, Oisin, who 'suffered' this process with me but who always wanted me to do and be better. He put things in perspective when I could not go on anymore. When I look back on all these years of hard work, he was always there.

Part I
Motherhood and culture

Introduction

Setting the contemporary scene

This study evolved as a response to societal/cultural and psychological changes faced by contemporary society. These changes are different from those in previous generations. As a psychotherapist, I began to encounter mothers who were not at the higher end of postnatal depression, but who presented with a certain maternal anxiety. Although this anxiety was a type of generalised anxiety disorder, it had the potential to progress into other types of anxiety. Some examples were: compulsive obsessive behaviours in the mother and/or treating/dealing with the baby, and agoraphobia, where the mother ceased to go out anywhere and remained at home with baby, for fear of not coping in public places. Many mothers I encountered also sought counselling for the simple reason that they found the transition to motherhood too overwhelming and could not put into words what they were feeling.

Not being able to 'put into words what we are feeling' is a common psychological experience. When applied to the transition to motherhood, it is a multi-layer event as some experiences are not recognised at a societal or cultural level. Mothers may feel lost, displaced, dissident in a space that does not acknowledge them. The words of Anita Diamant in the book, *The Red Tent* described this sentiment perfectly:

> Just as there is no warning for childbirth, there is no preparation for the sight of a first child. ... There should be a song for women to sing at this moment, or a prayer to recite. But perhaps there is none because there are no words strong enough to name the moment.
>
> (Diamant 1997, 269)

This quotation tries to conceptualise or even ritualise the enormous passage of giving birth into some kind of spiritual creative act or practice by showing how challenging this is even linguistically; how hard is to find the words. There is a difficulty in naming an experience if there is no language to acknowledge it.

Mothers who I encountered for years narrated existential fears and anxieties after child birth. They also experienced deep transformations to their social, psychological and interpersonal relationships. Their experiences needed to be conceptualised. They wanted to find an existential meaning to many questions that opened up after becoming a mother. Through these mothers, I began to understand that the maternal experiences of women following childbirth has been neglected in the non-depressed populations. Numerous studies have, and continue to concentrate on postpartum anxiety, stress and maternal anxiety during the transition to motherhood. Most of this work has concentrated on maternal depression from a biological and psychological framework, and also on the mother/infant interaction (Barlow 1997; Bernier *et al.* 2016; Emmanuel *et al.* 2011; Gauthier *et al.* 2010; Liamputtong 2007; Matthey 2010; 2011; Petrozzi and Gagliardi 2013; Garfield *et al.* 2016; Rallis *et al.* 2014; Santos *et al.* 2016; Sockol *et al.* 2014; Staneva *et al.* 2015). These studies also tended to evaluate different psychological therapies in the treatment and prevention of postnatal depression. Many studies have developed different quantitative instruments to measure maternal anxiety and depression in the pre- and postnatal period. There were, for example, studies that investigated quantitative instruments to measure the transition to motherhood in clinical settings.

At the time of my initial literature research, I found very few collections of qualitative data in the study of spirituality in the maternal transition. In 2010, an article was published in the *Journal of Nursing Management*, entitled: 'Being in Charge – New Mothers' Perceptions of Reflective Leadership and Motherhood' (Akerjordet 2010). This study investigated the importance of emotions as layers of meaning. It concluded that the transformation, growth and transition to motherhood is mediated by reflective self-acceptance, spirituality and increasing self-awareness. This article awakened my belief that it is important to understand what mothers considered to be meaningful emotions, desires and beliefs for their emotional adjustment. It also opened all kinds of questions about the view of women as integrated body/soul/mind beings passing through the unique transformation of becoming a mother. Many studies have been researched from the infant's perspective, and are so-called baby-centred. There was a lack of woman-centred studies: on how the mother needs to be supported and assisted through the liminal space of giving birth.

Many studies have investigated the neurobiological causes and the diverse biological changes that were likely to happen in pregnancy and during the postnatal period. The social/cultural and psychological studies on motherhood started after the second wave of feminism in the mid-twentieth century. From the 1960s onwards, and after the commercialisation of the pill and other contraceptives methods, the lives of women changed dramatically, with a trend to delay motherhood to latter years. The choice to become a mother is a complex one in which the life of the woman changes forever. These changes have provoked social/ economic and cultural shifts in developed Western countries. In the 1990s, studies began to concentrate on midwifery and the need for nurses to be educated in the spiritual dimension of childbirth. At the end of the twentieth century, a turn began to emerge for personal maternal experiences and narratives within the academia. Since 2001, birth and spirituality has also been increasingly researched from the nursing/midwifery framework.[1]

The importance of the psycho-spiritual dimensions of motherhood

The relationship between spirituality and motherhood has not been extensively researched, despite the fact that a growing body of scientific research suggests deep connections between religion, spirituality and both mental and physical health. Motherhood is a relatively new academic discipline and has always been considered 'private work', and a domain that did not have a 'voice' academically. For years, the pre- and postnatal periods have been researched within a biomedical model to improve the wellbeing of mothers and babies. Most of the maternal literature research studies on the process of the transition to motherhood included the constant change and transformation of redefining relationships, professional goals and self-identity. In 2005, a study on the spiritual awakening through the motherhood journey described the changes experienced by mothers as those of having achieved self-acceptance and expansion of consciousness (Miller and Athan 2005). The study recognises that spirituality is an essential and integral part of the mothering experience and that these descriptions are related to the transformation of the spiritual dimension of the self. It concludes that women who navigate this journey unassisted and unprepared are at a high risk of dysfunction.

Spirituality is subjective, intangible and multidimensional. There is little consensus regarding the number and content of the dimensions to sufficiently delineate it. The subjective dimension of spirituality also poses challenges in trying to conceptualise experiences that have unique and individual phenomenological qualities that may impact thoughts, behaviours, lifestyle and personality. A key factor in the definition of spirituality is the widespread need for humanity to search for meaning and purpose in life and consequently the construction of spiritual identity. This study understands the term spirituality as an inherent component of being human, but also acknowledges the difficulty of defining such a term. Spirituality is understood from an anthropological level as intrinsically part of human beings and as composed of physical, emotional and cognitive dimensions. Spiritual needs are as real as our need for love, food and shelter. Spirituality is a basic need, and a need that has been expressed since the beginning of time. The definition of spirituality better suited to this study is one that involves a person's beliefs, experiences and feelings about the self and important relationships. Indeed, spiritual identity has been defined as that dimension of self that addresses ultimate questions about the nature, purpose and meaning of life, resulting in behaviours that are consonant with the individual's core values (Kiesling *et al.* 2006).

Spirituality studies engage multidisciplinary and interdisciplinary fields. By researching motherhood through the academic discipline of spirituality, the whole person in the experience is investigated. In maternal health, many health problems are interrelated. Although some maternal physical issues are more visible, there are other invisible health needs. This shows the importance of a multidisciplinary and interdisciplinary study of spirituality when researching human experiences. Thus, researching an important human transition through the academic discipline of spirituality ensures that the 'full picture' is being looked at. Many questions began to emerge: what are the spiritual tools and qualities that we have? How do we use them in the transition to motherhood? Many research studies have shown the profound physical, cognitive and emotional changes that mothers undergo, but what about the spiritual changes? How is spirituality mediated in the transition to motherhood? What role does spirituality have in this transition? Can spiritual capacities help this transition? How might they be used by the mother? Does anything change spiritually for a woman once she becomes a mother?

With all these areas of enquiry, the need is for this study to concentrate on:

- The importance of identifying the academic interdisciplinary partners in the spirituality study.
- The importance of searching for spiritual skills/tools/capacities that can assist the mother in the transition.
- How these capacities are used by the mother.
- The spiritual changes or transformations in the lives of women once they become mothers.

Investigating these lines of inquiry seems relevant and significant to fill the gap of the spiritual dimension in the whole transition to motherhood in the current maternal literature.

The transition to motherhood is a unique experience and seems difficult to standardise. Societal attempts to polarise and express the transition to mother-hood in dichotomies may be a way of trying to standardise it. But motherhood resists such terms. I believe that maternal ambivalence has emerged out of these societal attempts to standardise. Postmodern parenting can be sadistically stress-ful and perfectionist. The deferment of childbearing, low natality rates in developed countries and the 'buying time approach', facilitated by assistive reproduction technology, can be the direct consequences of such ambivalence. It is not even about becoming a mother, as voluntary childlessness certainly reflects maternal ambivalence.

In 1935, a young mother using the nom de plume 'Ubique' (Latin for 'every-where') from Ballingate (Wicklow) in Ireland wrote a letter to *Nursery World* magazine in the United Kingdom (UK), expressing her feelings of isolation and loneliness:

> Can any mother help me? I live a very lonely life as I have no near neigh-bours. I cannot afford to buy a wireless. I adore reading, but with no library am very limited with books … I get so down and depressed after the chil-dren are in bed and I am alone in the house. I have had a rotten time, and been cruelly hurt, both physically and mentally, but I know it is bad to brood and breed hard thoughts and resentments. Can any reader suggest an

occupation that will intrigue me and exclude 'thinking' and cost nothing! A hard problem, I admit.

(Bailey 2007, 5)

Women from all over the country experiencing similar frustrations wrote back to her. A group of these mothers created an outlet for their life experiences (marriage life, children and friendships) by writing to each other and creating the Cooperative Correspondence Club (CCC). This secret magazine CCC continued until 1990, 55 years after the first issue was formulated.[2] Support and networking have always been crucial for mothers. Isolation and loneliness are probably the biggest enemies in any important life transition. The psyche tends to 'isolate' itself when an experience becomes in any way difficult. It is not a very beneficial survival mechanism. I have realised, through counselling mothers and interviewing them in research, that they sometimes become like 'veterans of war'. They find it hard to talk about the 'action' (maternal experiences) and become very secretive about their own struggles and feelings. The societal and cultural normalisation of maternal ambivalence would be much easier if there were a 'maternal agora' to engage deeply with the real experiences of the transition. I find it challenging to visualise this. The reality is that the technological revolution has in cyberspace monopolised the 'agora', and there is no way back from this. Mothers do not need to write to a magazine and wait for months to receive a postal letter. Comments in any maternal forums may be read by millions with a click. There is new-found freedom in being heard and acknowledged.

Back in 2013 I was surveying mothers for a study on stay-at-home mums. I posted a call to participate in a survey in maternal forums, and many mothers were ready to help me. Many wrote to me thanking me for researching such a theme. Mothers also asked me to consider them for any maternal research I might do in the future. I felt the response was overwhelming. They were eager to freely tell me their experiences. Some of them wrote me lengthy responses that I did not need for survey research, but they had the desire to tell me their 'maternal stories'. It was like entering a parallel universe. Mothers from all over the world at any time of the day are there to 'chat' and to 'engage'.

In postmodern times, mothers are deeply interested in maternal narratives and in validating and making meaning of their own experiences. In many cases, mothers do not feel free to talk about their maternal ambivalence and the array of feelings that this transition provokes: intense joy, love, lost, elation, happiness, sadness, frustration and much more. The light 'forces' in operation in the transition to motherhood are easily talked to but it is the opposite with the 'dark' forces, which exist within us. They are often denied, degraded and repressed. In motherhood, the Medea-mother archetype has the potential to 'shake' the very foundations of the societal and cultural maternal institution. I believe that the imbalance women have about caring for others and caring for themselves will always be at the core of maternal ambivalence. How much of this imbalance women can dare to recognise, and how conscious they become of their own power, will determine the reconciliation of these 'dark' forces. It is of vital importance to 'voice' and to try somehow to explore a linguistic framework in which spiritual capacities can be named and can make the mother more conscious in her own maternal transition.

Notes

1 A full maternal literature survey is researched in more detail, in Chapter 6.
2 In 2007, Jenna Bailey compiled all these stories in a book entitled, *Can Any Mother Help Me?*, published by Faber & Faber.

References

Akerjordet, K. 2010. 'Being in Charge – New Mothers' Perceptions of Reflective Leadership and Motherhood'. *Journal of Nursing Management* 18(4):409–417.

Bailey, J. 2007. *Can Any Mother Help Me?* London: Faber and Faber Limited.

Barlow, C. 1997. 'Mothering as a Psychological Experience: A Grounded Theory Exploration'. *Canadian Journal of Counselling* 31(3):232–237.

Bernier, A., Calkins, S., and Bell, M. 2016. 'Longitudinal Associations between the Quality of Mother–Infant Interactions and Brain Development across Infancy'. *Society for Research in Child Development* 30:1–16.

Diamant, A. 1997. *The Rent Tent.* New York: Picador Publishers.

Emmanuel, E., Creedy, D., St. John, W., Gamble, J., and Brown, C. 2008. 'Maternal Role Development following Childbirth among Australian Women'. *Journal of Advanced Nursing* 64:18–26.

Garfield, L., Mathews, H., and Janusek, L. 2016. 'Inflammatory and Epigenetic Pathways for Perinatal Depression'. *Biological Research for Nursing* 18(3):331–343.

Gauthier, L., Guay, F., Senecal, C., and Pierce, T. 2010. 'Women's Depressive Symptoms during the Transition to Motherhood: The Role of Competence, Relatedness, and Autonomy'. *Journal of Health Psychology* 8:1145–1156.

Kiesling, C., Montgomery, M., Sorell G., and Colwell, R. 2006. 'Identity and Spirituality: A Psychosocial Exploration of the Sense of Spiritual Self'. *Developmental Psychology* 42:1269–1277.

Liamputtong, P. 2007. 'When Giving Life Starts to Take the Life out of You: Women's Experiences of Depression after Childbirth'. *Midwifery* 23:77–91.

Matthey, S. 2010. 'Are We Overpathologising Motherhood?' *Journal of Affective Disorders* 120(1–3):263–266.

Matthey, S. 2011. 'Assessing the Experience of Motherhood: The Being a Mother Scale (BaM-13)'. *Journal of Affective Disorders* 128(1–2):142–152.

Miller, L., and Athan, A. 2005. 'Spiritual Awakening through the Motherhood Journey'. *Journal of the Association for Research on Mothering* 7(1):17–31.

Petrozzi, A., and Gagliardi, L. 2013. 'Anxious and Depressive Components of Edinburgh Postnatal Depression Scale in Maternal Postpartum Psychological Problems'. *Journal of Perinatal Medicine* 41(4):343–348.

Rallis, S., Skouteris, H., McCabe, M., and Milgrom, J. 2014. 'The Transition to Motherhood: Towards a Broader Understanding of Perinatal Distress'. *Women Birth* 27(1):68–71.

Santos, H., Yang, Q., Docherty, S., White-Traut, R., and Holditch-Davis, D. 2016. 'Relationship of Maternal Psychological Distress Classes to Later Mother-Infant Interaction,

Home Environment, and Infant Development in Preterm Infants'. *Research in Nursing and Health* 39(3):175–186.

Sockol, L., Epperson, C., and Barber, J. 2014. 'Relationship between Maternal Attitudes and Symptoms of Depression and Anxiety among Pregnant and Postpartum First-Time Mothers'. *Archives of Women's Mental Health* 17(3):199–212.

Staneva, A., Bogossian, F., and Wittkowski, A. 2015. 'The Experience of Psychological Distress, Depression, and Anxiety during Pregnancy: A Meta-Synthesis of Qualitative Research'. *Midwifery* 31(6):563–573.

1 Historical, cultural and psychological perspectives on motherhood

Historical perspectives on motherhood

Motherhood through the centuries

Throughout history, the status of the mother and generally the role of women in society has changed continuously depending on the specific cultural, social and political contexts. Much can be learned from reviewing motherhood through the centuries. The needs and culture of a specific civilisation at any point in history have influenced how the maternal role is socially constructed and understood. Motherhood and marriage have been highly valued and prominent expectations for women throughout the centuries, with societies being structured around the family unit.

Women's primary duties were usually to bear children and take care of the household. Often ancient societies worshipped multiple goddesses of motherhood and fertility, and evidence of mother goddess worship has been found from as early as 24,000 BCE. Mother goddesses were often assimilated into later belief systems. Isis was an Egyptian goddess of motherhood, along with Inanna, a Mesopotamian goddess of nature and fertility. Later on, Isis and Inanna were assimilated into the Greek belief system, under the names of Aphrodite/Demeter/Astarte, thus extending mother worship in Europe (Pomeroy 1991).

The earliest agricultural societies (CE 12,000 to CE 500) in Western Asia, Egypt and the Indus Valley (modern Iran and Pakistan) raised children in a communal way. This Neolithic Revolution, which started 12,000 years ago, was a traditional hunter-gatherer society. The production of agricultural surpluses gave way to the emergence of ancient civilisations which remained mainly agricultural. The first ancient civilisations began to appear between approximately 5000 BCE and 3500 BCE in Mesopotamia and Egypt. Egyptian women enjoyed a higher status than women elsewhere in the ancient world. Some were educated property owners and were allowed to keep inheritance (Tyldesley 1984). Mothers in Egypt tended to be affectionate and nurturing, ensuring that their children had a happy childhood (Cantarella 1987).

By contrast, in Roman times (CE 55 to CE 122) fathers had absolute rights over their children. A Roman woman could be married either *in manu* (into her husband's hands, in which case he owned and controlled her property) or *sine manu*, in which case she remained under the control of her father but could become legally independent after bearing three children. In Roman societies most mothers were strict disciplinarians who determined the children's future roles in society. Although women had no political rights, they were often believed to exert power behind the scenes through their husband or son (Bradley 1991).

Once Christianity had become the dominant religion in the Roman Empire, by the fifth century CE, women's roles in Western society changed. By CE 476, the last Roman Emperor was deposed, which saw the beginning a new era – the Middle Ages, or Medieval period. In the early Christian Church, women were treated equally to men and could assume leadership roles. This status changed in the Early Middle Ages (CE 500 to CE 1000), when much of European society was predominantly formed by Christian influences. The patriarchal and hierarchical organisation of Medieval times influenced motherhood. Major religions, such as Catholicism, Judaism and Islam, became patriarchal. It was at this time (CE 661 to CE 750) that Islam also spread into some parts of Europe and North Africa, during the Umayyad Caliphate. Medieval families usually had only two to three children who survived into adulthood, due to high infant mortality. Human life expectancy was approximately 30–35 years on average, but depended on the geographical location, and few records are available (Atkinson 1991).

In the period from 1000–1500, a transition began to take place between the ancient and modern worlds. Societies were becoming more complex, and urbanised commerce and industry were growing. Improved medical knowledge on the approach to pregnancy and childbirth coexisted with superstitious and religious beliefs. A collection of texts called *The Trotula* appeared in Italy in the eleventh and twelfth centuries, outlining female health topics such as menstruation, fertility, pregnancy and childbirth (Green 2001). Some women owned their own property and were abbesses in charge of monasteries, but the female division of labour and cultural female roles generally remained the same as in previous eras. Since the family's power often relied on their children's upbringing, women could obtain power by raising strong boys and gentle girls (Gies and Gies 1987).

Many events contributed to the decline of the Middle Ages. The Black Death ravaged Europe in 1347, killing millions and destroying the feudal system, which provided the basis for society in Medieval times. The capture of Constantinople in 1453 by the Ottoman Empire, ended the Eastern Roman Empire. The colonisation of 'The Americas' in 1492, the widespread use of gunpowder and the expulsion of Muslim and Jew inhabitants in Europe in 1499, also contributed to the decline of the Late Medieval period and the Great Western European transformation into the Early Modern period. The cultural movement of the Renaissance deeply influenced this European change, and its intellectual life, from the fourteenth to the seventeenth century (Armstrong 2001).

In the period from 1500–1800, motherhood became a valued institution of great significance, with motherhood and politics becoming intertwined. In many societies, mothers were defined by their relationships with their children and so they stayed in the home and raised them according to the cultural and political expectations. Of sixteenth-century England, Robert Filmer wrote: 'the family is the essence and a microcosm of the state' (Sommerville 1991). Western ideology developed a social and political construct based on gendered hierarchical relationships between men and women. Women were legally defined as *femme covert*, which meant that all legal and political matters were conducted by their husbands. If women were unmarried, they were represented legally and socially by their fathers, and in this way, the state was connected and linked through family and motherhood. Women's existence was validated by the act of becoming mothers (Aughterson 1995).

From 1500–1750, there was very little knowledge about how reproduction worked, and the role that women played in conception. Many women herbalists were killed in this period because they had extensive knowledge of contraceptives and abortifacients, and so could assist women in managing their fertility. Some scholars argue that this was motivated by the desire of male doctors to take control of female fertility (Lerner 1993).

The Enlightenment (1620–1780) and the beginning of the Scientific Revolution marked one of the biggest transformations in the Early Modern period. French historians place the Enlightenment between 1715 and 1789, with the start of the French Revolution. Others place it in 1620, with the advent of the Scientific Revolution. Nevertheless, this period is fundamental in the emergence of modern sciences such as mathematics, physics, astronomy, biology and chemistry. The French Revolution and the Enlightenment encouraged women to become educators and promote organisations on proper child rearing (Allen 2005). During the Enlightenment, men and women spent hours discoursing over political and social issues, while women played an important part by hosting salons, where these debates took place. The first of these salons was in the *Hôtel de Rambouillet* in Paris, whose hostess, Catherine de Vivonne, Marquise de Rambouillet (1588–1665), remained a key figure of this literary movement. These social groups extended to other European capitals such as London, Vienna, Rome, Copenhagen and Berlin (Abrams 2002).

A new ideology of motherhood emerged from the philosophy of the Enlightenment, whose thinkers, after all, emphasised a moral and well-educated population as the foundation of the home, the family and society. Many philosophers circulated among these groups, including Jean-Jacques Rousseau, who changed ideas about motherhood in France. Rousseau's ideas gained popularity and became known as the 'Cult of Motherhood', whereby he stressed the importance of the mother as the primary caretaker and nurturer of her child (Rousseau 2007).

Across the Atlantic, the American Revolution (1775–1783) also influenced motherhood. The political role of women in the early American Republic was viewed as that of mothers who were raising future republican citizens. If a republic was to succeed, women must be schooled so that they could, in turn, teach their children. The first American female academies were founded in the 1790s. A Republican Motherhood ideal[1] was born out of women's traditional, civic duty to raise the next generation (Kerber 1980). Thus, women felt they needed to be better educated in order to serve their country. Republican Motherhood was the transitional paradigm between the colonial good wife and the nineteenth-century ideal of a 'True Woman', who was pious, pure, submissive and domestic (Lindley 1996). True Womanhood was also referred to as the 'Cult of Domesticity', in which women's choices for work, education and opinions were 'privatised'. Women should remain away from the public sphere and were seen as better suited to parenting. This culture of domesticity, or Cult of True Womanhood, was the value system endorsed by the upper and middle classes during the nineteenth century in the United States (US) and the UK. The result of this value system was the support of a gendered vision of citizenship that emphasised women's domesticity.

In the period from 1800–1900, mothers' roles changed dramatically and consolidated into the modern understanding of gender, which has only been successfully challenged in the latter half of the twentieth century. The gender construction was based on Republican Motherhood, True Womanhood, the Cult of Motherhood (French movement) and the Victorian notions of how women belonged to the private sphere of the home (Boyer 2000). In the eighteenth and nineteenth centuries, the Industrial Revolution took place in Europe, changing the traditional family economy into the family wage economy. Need for wages changed work patterns of women and children, depending on whether they were single, married or childbearing. The impact of this revolution varied between the different socioeconomic classes. Working-class mothers and young girls worked in textile factories and in domestic service (Tilly and Scott 1989).

Scientific knowledge was rapidly advancing and helped to better elucidate the conception process. Karl Ernst von Baer discovered the mammalian ovum in 1827, and in 1928, Edgar Allen discovered the human ovum. The fusion of spermatozoa with ova (of a starfish) was observed by Oskar Hertwig in 1876 (Cobb 2012). Thus, the seeds of a scientific approach to mothering were set down in this period. Women began to lose active participation in childbirth, and men, with their surgical tools, gained power over the midwives, thus becoming the authority on childbirth (Epstein 2010).

From 1900, major world events, especially World War I (WWI) and World War II (WWII), altered the perceptions of motherhood in the Europe and the US. During the war eras, women entered the labour force. Mothers were given medals, financial support and day-care facilities for their children. Women supported the military effort as nurses, female military auxiliaries, ambulance drivers, farm workers and factory labourers (Grayzel 2002). Florence Nightingale (1820–1910) was a precursor for war work and the founder of modern nursing. By 1920, most women in Western countries had been granted the right to vote. During the period between WWI and WWII, medicine, psychology and other sciences increased. Mothers in Europe started to lose their agency, as new professionals roles in medicine and psychology increased, and the role holders were considered the experts. Hospital birthing expanded, replaced home birthing, and became highly medicalised (Apple 2006).

In the period between 1945 and 1965, the icons of motherhood changed again. Once the war ended, women were encouraged to fulfil their truest destiny of producing children and being homemakers. In the US, that condition was described by Betty Friedan as the 'feminine mystique' (Friedan 1963). The publication of this title enabled millions of women to see how the roles they fulfilled in society as wives and mothers were not the only roles they could achieve in life. It is important to note that the data for this research was gathered from upper middle-class white mothers, who had sympathies with Friedan's views. Marginalised or non-white mothers failed to fit into this 'feminine mystique' analysis, either culturally, politically, socially or economically (Horowitz 1998).

This historical review, although brief, can elucidate social, cultural and economical maternal patterns visible through the centuries. Women were responsible for the raising of children in accordance with the religious, philosophical, cultural beliefs of the particular society in which they lived. It was not until the end of the 1960s that drastic social changes started happening in Western society. These social changes deconstructed many practices of motherhood and also gave raise others. By the end of the twentieth century, new trends and perceptions of motherhood began to emerge and these still influence mothers today.

Motherhood in the twenty-first century

A new trend came about in the early 1990s called 'intensive mothering' (also known as the 'new momism') and it has survived until the present day. Most women in their 30s and 40s are culturally influenced by this model of motherhood. The term 'intensive mothering' was first coined by Sharon Hays to refer to a movement which started in North America in the 1980s (Hays 1998a). She believes that the purpose of intensive mothering is a re-domestication of women, many of whom were becoming well educated and entering the marketplace. Simultaneously, the media also overflowed with new information on maternal options for the new lifestyle, with huge marketing campaigns on what it was to be a good mother. All types of baby products from the right buggy, the right toys and the 'proper' food were strategically advertised in these campaigns to educate mothers. A good mother knew and was aware of every single thing that benefited the physical and psychological development of the child (Hays 1998b). These campaigns served the consumer society. The relationship between consumerism and motherhood is an important subject. The meaning of this consumeristic trend is about micromanaging every single aspect of the child's development, and it is intrinsically related to 'intensive mothering'.

Many studies have demonstrated how 'intensive mothering' is the current maternal philosophy from which especially upper middle-class women operate (McMahon 1995; Choi *et al.* 2005; Miller 2005; Petrassi 2012; Ennis 2014). Western women, regardless of ethnicity, race, social class, religion and employment status, are enchanted by the expectations of intensive mothering. It has been noted that middle and upper middle-class mothers are most likely to engage in this practice to the extreme (Hays 1998b). Motherhood today is clearly influenced by consumerism and capitalism, and this has also complicated expectations and identities of motherhood and mothering in the last two decades.

The core belief of intensive mothering, in its own right, is that children need and require constant nurturing by their biological mothers, who are primarily responsible for meeting four primary needs: physical, emotional, spiritual and social. Therefore, mothers must rely on experts to guide them and they must invest large amounts of time and energy in their children. This way, mothers consider mothering more important than paid work (O'Reilly 2010). Thus, time, energy, expertise and constancy are the core beliefs of this ideology.

The impossible standards of intensive mothering have been criticised and challenged. Recently, to celebrate the twentieth anniversary of Sharon Hays' book, *The Cultural Contradictions of Motherhood*, a new publication on 'intensive mothering' was published by Demeter Press (Ennis 2014). The scholars who contributed to the book raised the question of why we are still engaging in intensive motherhood, in a world where independence is encouraged. Such an ideology not only undermines mothers and de-humanises them, but also creates a constant dichotomy and battle between them.

In 1990, Nina Darnton, in an article for *Newsweek* magazine, coined the phrase: 'mummy wars' to describe the battle between paid, working mothers and stay-at-home mothers. The 'mummy wars' arise from the rivalry between women to become a 'good mother' or the 'best mother of all mothers' (Douglas and Meredith 2005). Indeed, Irigaray (1985a) believes that the core of the patriarchal system relies on 'making it impossible for women to love each other'.

Intensive mothering is just another way in which cultural ambivalence arises from the needs of the marketplace. In the twenty-first century, there is pressure to conform to market standards of mothering, and mothers are under constant pressure to make tough choices around caring, work, autonomy and power. Mothers embody the economic and cultural ambivalence of society. Since the Industrial Revolution, a cultural model of a rationalised market society has come to coexist in tension with the cultural model of intensive mothering (Hays 1998b).

Many mothers are reacting to this cultural ambivalence and trying to create an identity for their unique style of mothering. Personal maternal narratives have become popular – memoirs, books, blogs – and are challenging intensive mothering (Sotirin 2010). These unique maternal narratives from all types of mothers (marginalised, women of colour, etc.) are showing that intensive mothering is a narrowed, controlled and restricted way to encapsulate the complex experiences of parenting.

Motherhood and feminism

Feminism approaches the study of mothering from the perspective of women's desires, children's needs and the power structures in the family and society as a whole. It challenges common assumptions about the domestication of women.

In the UK, by the nineteenth century, the seeds of first-wave feminism were planted by women's advocates such as Mary Wollstonecraft, Frances Wright and Harriet Martineau. They were accused of disrupting the natural order of things and challenged the ideal of the Cult of True Womanhood/Domesticity. These advocates endorsed the New Woman, feminist ideal that profoundly influenced feminism well into the twentieth century (Patterson 2008). British-American writer Henry James popularised the term 'New Woman' to describe feminist, educated, independent career women in Europe and the US (Stevens 2008).

The New Woman is frequently associated with the suffrage movement. In the US, Margaret Fuller is considered by some as the first major feminist. In 1845, she published her feminist classic, *Woman in the Nineteenth Century*, a book profoundly affecting the women's rights movement, which formally began at the Seneca Falls Convention, New York, three years later (1848). This was the first women's rights convention and was established to discuss the social, civil and religious condition and rights of women, influencing the first wave of feminism (Ford 2008). Motherhood was clearly not an issue with this first wave of feminists, whose concerns were political – in particular, the right to vote. It was not until the 1960s, with second-wave feminism, that motherhood was addressed.

Feminist thinking about maternity began in the early 1960s and is characterised by diverse movements within the same second wave of feminism (from the 1960s until the early 1990s). Early feminists in this period took a radical approach to uncovering the oppression of motherhood in society. Generally, maternity was presented as a negative experience. Main figures during this period included Simone de Beauvoir, Shulamith Firestone, Kate Millet and Betty Friedan. They fought hard to destroy narrow gendered constructions of motherhood. The release of new contraceptive methods, such as the birth control pill (early 1960s), meant that many of these young feminists could avoid motherhood. They were concerned with a woman's right to control her fertility, her access to childcare and her freedom to choose any lifestyle (Millet 1970). They viewed biology as inherently oppressive for all women and presented maternity as a set and immutable role (de Beauvoir 1949; Firestone 1970). For these theorists, maternity cannot be revised: it must be 'avoided' or 'sidestepped'. Friedan did not propose a new view of maternity, but a 'scape' from the domestic realm by means of education and employment (Friedan 1963).

The second wave of feminism has been accused of being 'anti-mother' in the public discourse and in the media. Although some feminists proposed a 'philosophy of evacuation', and generally viewed motherhood as an oppressive patriarchal institution (Allen 1986), other feminist writings and activists explored mothering differently. In the mid-1970s, attempts to recover, reclaim and revise maternity were begun by feminists such as Adrienne Rich, Nancy Chodorow, Dorothy Dinnerstein and Sara Ruddick in the US; Mary O'Brien and Juliet Mitchell in the UK; and Luce Irigaray, Helene Cixous and Julia Kristeva in France.

Adrienne Rich made an important distinction: she tried to uncover the 'institution of motherhood' (Rich 1976) as a different entity from the 'mothering experience'. For her, the institution was patriarchal, male defined, controlling and oppressive to women, while the mothering experience of women was female defined and empowering. In summary, Rich tried to make a distinction between 'motherhood' as an institution and 'mothering' as the maternal experience. She argued for a reconciliation of motherhood as a source of strength to women.

Chodorow and Dinnerstein's work drew on Freudian psychoanalysis. They both argued that patriarchy and misogyny are rooted in women's monopoly over childrearing. Chodorow critiques how the mother is almost entirely made responsible for the child's development and this is what reproduces the gender differences of patriarchy (Chodorow 1978). Dinnerstein believed that only a radical shift in gender roles could fight the deep resistance to change. She blamed the 'defensive psychological functions' that traditional childrearing still serves to society as a whole. As long as childhood is ruled by the mother alone, the child will take revenge on her and on her surrogate, Mother Nature. She offered a deep study on the unconscious and complex arrangement of gender in society and highlighted the ambivalent relationship women have with owning their own power. She believed that the powerful rage of feminism came from the unconscious private griefs that women have endured through centuries (Dinnerstein 1976).

Ruddick is probably, one of the most important feminist philosophers in second-wave feminism. For her, maternal practice involved responding to the tripartite demands of children: to preserve their life, to help with their growth and to implant them with skills to become acceptable within a community. The way the mother reflects, judges and deals with her emotions which are evoked in relation to these demands, is what she calls 'maternal thinking' (Ruddick 1989). Her contribution transformed the earlier feminism of motherhood, in which maternity and domestic labour were understood as non-productive and without value. She articulated maternal values necessary for maternal practice, thus revaluing maternity without retreating to biology, essentialism or romanticism.

In the UK, Juliet Mitchell and Mary O'Brien were the main contributors to feminism and motherhood in this era. In the 1970s and 1980s, many feminists believed in the importance of 'taking back control of the birth process', as it had become dominated by men in the medical profession (Kinser 2010). O'Brien was concerned with the biological base of women's reproductive labour as creative. She was not interested in the whole ideology and practice of gender. Her theories mark a shift from the course of the female biology of early second-wave feminists. Her criticism of de Beauvoir was for not recognising the material connection between women and reproduction, or the link between reproductive labour and creative labour. She offered a unique feminist analysis of female and male reproductive processes and experiences, and stressed women's experiences and the vulnerability of men's position in the process of reproduction. She was able to explain masculine and feminine experiences as a result of actual difference in reproductive praxis and bodily experience, making a distinction between the male and the female reproductive consciousness. She believed that male reproductive consciousness arising from experiences of the body may have initiated patriarchy as an institution that influences gender and power. Female reproductive consciousness, on the other hand, is a born act of woman's labour, which confirms genetic coherence and species continuity. These reproductive processes were called the dialectics of reproduction. She believed in the stand-point of women, as Marx had assumed the standpoint of the proletariat. She coined the expression 'malestream', in reference to traditional, mainstream polit-ical and philosophical Western thought. Her work has been very important in rethinking not only reproduction, but social life/policy, leadership, sexuality, fatherhood and the relation of the public and the private. She challenged women to think beyond seeking integration into the productive sphere and believed that liberation also depends on the reintegration of men, on equal terms, into the reproductive process (O'Brien 1981).

Also, at this time, feminism turned to psychoanalysis as the best starting point from which to describe femininity and how it is produced. The first serious engagement with Freud, from a feminist perspective, was theorised by Juliet Mitchell, who belongs to the Freudian psychoanalytic feminism movement and is thus concerned with the psychic production of male dominance and the devel-opment of gendered subjects in societies where women are left solely respons-ible for mothering and rearing children. She reconciled psychoanalysis and feminism at a time when it was considered incompatible, feeling that feminists had rejected the wrong Freud – a maligned/misogynist figure based on de Beau-voir's writings.

Her feminism critique involved a 'literalisation programme' to bring Freudian ideas into feminism. She viewed Freud's views on gender as a reflection of the patriarchal culture in which he lived. In her most famous book, *Psychoanalysis and Feminism: Freud, Reich, Laing and Women*, she devoted her thesis on how Marxism may provide a model in which non-patriarchal structures of engendered children can happen. She believed that removing the 'family phantasy' of the Oedipus complex from the child's development can result in liberating women from the gender roles that have been assigned to them since childhood (Mitchell 1974). She opened a door in the feminist debate on Freud and gender and made a considerable contribution to reconciling psychoanalysis and feminism.

In France, the women's liberation movement emerged after the student and worker revolt of May 1968. *Psychoanalyse et Politique* (Psychoanalysis and Pol-itics) was a group formed at this time. French feminists such as Irigaray (1985a), Kristeva (1986) and Cixous (1975) emerged out of this group. They were inter-ested in Lacanian psychoanalysis and how it impacts on gendered identity, lan-guage and maternal subjectivity. Lacan's rereading of Freud emphasises an interpretation of language and the symbolic in order to create a gendered subjectivity.

In his seminar, 'On Feminine Sexuality, the Limits of Love and Knowledge',[2] he points out:

> Freud argues that there is no libido other than masculine. Meaning what? Other than that a whole field, which is hardly negligible, is thereby ignored.

This is the field of all those beings who take on the status of the woman – if, indeed, this being takes on anything whatsoever of her fate.

(Lacan 1985, 151)

In the 1990s, feminist scholars became involved in debates about essentialism. Third-wave, maternal feminists such as Susan Maushart believe that second-wave feminism washed over motherhood and that women's lives have changed dramatically from the 'tranquillised' empty lives that Friedan described, to those of 'juggling' multiple expectations and responsibilities. Thus, the mothering experience has become more complex (Maushart 1999). Studies on 'real' maternal lives were published at this time. They were unapologetic maternal autobiographies relating everyday motherhood experiences. These groundbreaking books, published in the 1990s, include: Marni Jackson's: *The Mother Zone: Love, Sex and Laundry in the Modern Family* (1992); Phyllis Burke and Debbie Kwan's: *Family Values: Two Moms and Their Son* (1993); Annie Lamott's: *Operating Instructions: A Journal of My Son's First Year* (1994); Louise Erdrich's: *The Blue Jay's Dance: A Birth Year* (1995); and Jane Lazarre's: *Beyond the Whiteness of Whiteness: Memoir of a White Mother of Black Sons* (1996). They showed that women often experience isolation, lack of support and lack of preparation for the demands of caring for a baby (Brown *et al.* 1994).

There was a whole new deconstruction of gender in third-wave feminism, which again impacted on the understanding of becoming a mother. Third-wave feminism challenged the assumptions of second-wave, feminism ethnocentric studies in relation to classed experiences, histories of enslavement, colonisation and racism. These new maternal autobiographies related motherhood through various socioeconomic classes, racial, ethnic and sexual identities. The main focus of third-wave feminism in relationship to motherhood was: the issues of power related to the status of mothers in society, with particular reference to their economic resources, and also the issue of labour for mothers, and the vulnerable position of taking most of the unpaid caring work in the world in a monetised society. Issues of cultural biases imposed on mothers to reach unattainable goals in being a 'good mother' are central to third-wave feminism. The issue of pre- and postnatal health in the lives of the mothers and their children came to the fore during this time. Finally, issues of family planning and reproductive control, by which women are fighting for the right of their bodies' integrity in motherhood, are very much part of this third movement (Jetter *et al.* 1997).

Third-wave research on feminism and mothering became more complex than second-wave feminism. In 2006, the *Journal of the Association for Research on Mothering* published an edition on the theme of Mothering and Feminism. Maternal feminist scholars in the third wave felt the need to name the oppressive and empowering aspects of maternity and the complex relationship between the two. Third-wave feminism thought perceived the nature of maternity as active, complex and changeable under the influence of poststructuralism and postmodernism (Jeremiah 2006). Many third-wave feminists have proposed that the 'maternal experience' is not separable from its construction, and conceive mothering as active, relational and transformative. Maternal activity is defined by the acts that the mother performs in relation to the needs of the other. Questions of ethics, choice, care and moral decisions are inevitably present for mothers.

Third-wave, postmodern feminist literature approaches contemporary mothering practices as a 'deconstruction' of traditional maternal subjectivity (Waugh 1989) and third-wave women's personal, maternal writings tend to 'explore different modes of relational identity' (Waugh 1989). For them, maternal subjectivity is not static, but rather in process, constantly constructed or 'performed'. It is possible for these theorists to speak of 'maternal subjectivities' as a key difference amongst women (Butler 2000). Thus, maternal personal narratives are important in this period. Some critical studies have been published in the last decade: *Third Wave Feminism: A Critical Exploration*, by Gillis *et al.* (2007) and 'Third Wave Feminism, Motherhood and the Future of Feminist Legal Theory', by Crawford (2011). These critiques exposed that some of the personal narratives on fertility and motherhood produced by third-wave feminism have contributed to enhancing the mythology of motherhood that second-wave feminism had tried to destroy. Third-wave feminists loudly proclaimed their difference from feminists who had come before, but in doing so, they over-emphasised and even elevated women's reproductive achievements over others. Most of these third-wave feminist maternal writings were written in the first-person, often recounting the journey towards motherhood as a rite of passage. Three representative examples of such milestone narrative books from this period are: Rebecca Walker's *Baby Love* (2007), Evelyn McDonnell's *Mama Rama* (2007) and Peggy Orenstein's *Waiting for Daisy* (2007).

However, in reality, third-wave feminists construct a framework which permits simultaneous critique and embracing of motherhood (Crawford 2011). These maternal narratives can also challenge the traditional notions of knowledge, based on the dichotomy and hierarchical spheres of object/subject (Jeremiah 2002). The 'subjectivities' expressed in the contemporary maternal narratives are characterised by relationality and bodiliness, and may be seen as the cornerstone of social, economic and political transformations for mothers (Chandler 1998). The empowerment of mothers in these lived realities seems the main focus of third-wave feminism. By contrast, silence contributes to the loss of power and authority which results in loss of confidence, feelings of blame, guilt and conflicting thoughts. Guilt is certainly widespread and striking and is an indicator of the privatised nature of the present pursuit of balance, and the privatised nature of disappointment that mothers alone cannot always achieve (Pocock 2001). Maternal guilt is so powerful and common that a modern study, *Maternal Guilt: The Early Emotional Experiences of First-time Mothers*, by LeBeau (2013), exposes existential phenomenological experiences of guilt, and how they affect maternal relationships with others and the world. Normally, these guilt experiences become so complex that they are difficult to talk about. They also have the double bind of defensive and denial societal mechanisms.

Maternal ambivalence is the result of such feelings, and the reluctance of society to acknowledge this perpetuates the process.

In the last ten years, the internet has facilitated the creation of a global community of feminists, who use it both for discussion and activism (Munro 2013). The fourth-wave feminists have been described as 'tech-savvy and gender-sophisticated with their blogs, twitter campaigns and online media' (Baumgardner 2011). From the perspective of a psychoanalytic feminism, in the fourth wave, women turned towards spiritual concerns about the planet and all its beings, putting themselves in the service of the world, ecology and the downtrodden (Kimble 2009).

This lived, narrative creation process in cyberspace as a definite empowerment for mothers to engage in social and global change (O'Reilly 2011). It is a counter narrative to the classical social/historical narrative and seeks 'to fashion a mode of mothering that affords and affirms maternal agency, authority, autonomy and authenticity and which confers and confirms power to and for mothers' (O'Reilly 2004). Canadian Professor Andrea O'Reilly, expert on motherhood studies, believes that second-wave feminism presented motherhood as an oppressed institution and third-wave feminism romanticised the institution. She asserts that in fourth-wave feminism, mothers need a movement and theory of their own. Thus, she has created such a movement by the creation of a 'matricentric feminism'.

In May 2015, in a talk presented at the Motherhood and Culture conference in Maynooth University, Ireland entitled: 'Ain't I a Feminist? Matricentric Feminism, Feminist Mamas, and Why Mothers Need a Feminist Movement/Theory of their Own', O'Reilly raised the challenge:

> Significantly, during the second wave, when white women were rightly challenged for their white bias and privilege, they recognised the need for change though they were not themselves racialised women. So the present researcher is left still asking questions: Why are non-mother feminists not capable of doing the same for mothers today? Why are non-mothers unable to appreciate and respond to the demands of inclusion made by mothers as white women did for racialised women in the early years of the second wave? Why is motherhood not acknowledged as a subject position in constituting gendered identities? Why do we not see maternity as an interlocking structure of oppression, as we do with race and class, and include it in our gendered analysis of oppression and resistance? Why do we not recognize mothers' specific perspective as we do for other women whether they are queer, working-class, racialised, etc? Why doesn't motherhood count or matter?[3]

Feminist mothering studies seek to demonstrate that even within the patriarchal institution of motherhood, empowered mothers can 'explore and cultivate their own agency' (Green 2004) and 'consciously resist the restrictions placed on them' (Horowitz 2004), by 'seeing themselves as agents in control of their own life, rather than victims' (Ross 1995).

Thus, the nature of autonomy in the future is in question. Autonomy is related to agency and asserts that mothers need to be self-sufficient, financially and otherwise (Maushart 1999) Women's relationship with wealth will be paramount for mothers to care for their children or to be able to pay for childcare. Women's wealth involves material, social, psychological and spiritual dimensions (Ross and Purcell 2004).

Autonomy, authenticity, authority and agency are the cornerstones in the social, financial and political situations in which mothers often find themselves. Authenticity is a core dimension of spiritual growth and the spiritual capacity for self-reflection. This spiritual capacity can empower mothers to undertake sincere, inner exploration of their needs and also the needs of their children. Authenticity is the ability of the mother to be truthful and assertive with herself. This is quite difficult for mothers in Western culture, as they are encouraged to hide behind a 'mask of motherhood' (Maushart 1999). It is often the case that women do not speak the truth about what they know and fail to face challenges that threaten their current position. This conundrum will be at the core of motherhood and mothering theorising in the future.

Egalitarian partnership in the family, equal and integral parenting, sharing housework and childcare all need to be part of a fourth-wave maternal movement (Middleton 2006). The economics of motherhood and mother care-work were exposed with the publication of journalist Ann Crittenden's *The Price of Motherhood* (2001). The economic disadvantages of mothers as caregivers remain the unfinished business of the feminist movement. In the Western world, though women have entered the labour force, they still do most of the work of caring for children and are penalised by what Crittenden called the 'mommy tax'. Thus, mothers are at a much higher risk of poverty and financial hardship.

Crittenden (2001) and Naomi Wolf (2003) cofounded the organisation Mothers Ought to Have Equal Rights (MOTHERS) as a 'grassroots initiative seeking to improve caregivers' economy by calling attention to their essential contribution to the economy and to society' (Hewett 2006, 37).

Gender-divided 'parenting' and 'paid work' realities show how 'postfeminist' culture continues to devalue 'women's work'. These realities make the maternal transition very difficult for many mothers. Numerous studies and articles have analysed this dilemma (McDonough 2006; Turnbull 2006; Linker 2006). Feminists' agenda for change included the financial, social, cultural and spiritual empowerment of mothers. This empowerment has its intricacies. The feminism tactic of empowerment has served women for centuries. In any patriarchal culture, women can access power if it is justified by the children/family wellbeing. Real power cannot be achieved or defined solely as, and about, children/family (O'Reilly 2006).

This challenge is a difficult one. The waves of feminism are like surfing: they peak and then go down, and women (unsupported and unassisted) have to be careful not to drown with them. Women need to dare, without the 'system's' approval or support, to reconstruct and restructure an inner and outer change with their own relationship with empowerment.

The ancient great myth of Demeter and Persephone elucidated how children are best served by empowered mothers. Demeter is able to save her daughter because she is a powerful goddess who can make winter permanent and destroy humankind. Demeter possesses qualities, resources and strength that mothers often lack to protect their children, particularly daughters (Smith 2003). Crittenden argues that depriving mothers of an income and influence of their own is harmful to children, and a recipe for economic backwardness. When a culture devalues and enslaves the mother, she cannot be like Demeter and protect her daughter (Crittenden 2001).

Demeter's maternal empowerment is shown in the resources and strength in her inner self. In talking to Persephone, she said:

> Do not be afraid: I know of your hate. ... Do not think I require you back as you were, I know you are changed. And I too, daughter ... I also am changed. I embrace all of you, daughter, the change and the hate.
>
> (Downing 1994, 159)

The social-cultural constructions, often, do not allow for integration or an 'embrace' of the different aspects of motherhood. It is important to reveal such constructions in order to comprehend the depth in which the institution of motherhood is embedded.

The cultural milieu of motherhood

As seen above, the sociocultural constructions of motherhood need to be understood from the dynamic process of historical and societal evolution that is taking place in everyday interactions and actions. Sociocultural influences are ideological constructs that are established, adopted and institutionalised in culture within a historical framework. Rules and behaviours will follow this process frequently in a stable and immutable norm, profoundly influencing the perception of motherhood (Parton 2008). In order to understand the institution of motherhood, it is necessary to study both the object itself and the systems of knowledge that produced it.

When views about a certain identity are institutionalised and dominant in the sociocultural construction of truth, the individuals concerned will often engage in behaviour that reinforces such an identity to self and others (Snow and Anderson 1987). Thus, many women do not operate from their true selves as women, but 'as socially constructed selves, as mothers' (Tardy 2000). These 'constructed selves' change and mould, depending on the dominant political and economic ideology at any given time in history. One exception is the invariable way in which motherhood has been considered an 'idealised role' for women. This has become particularly strong as an ideological trend in the twenty-first century, as the construct of 'intensive mothering' shows. In idealisation, the feeling of love for a role, is distorted and unrealistic (Dally 1983).

The concept of 'too-good mothering' has been making headlines in the media for a long time. It refers to mothers whose lives are 'on hold', or their needs are replaced completely, by those of their children. Movie stars and singers are a good example of how the media have used this 'intensive mothering' ideal to portray an image of the archetypal, nurturing and universal mother. These stars make it look very easy to have six or seven children, look beautiful and be self-sacrificing. However, there is a strong competitive and narcissistic undercurrent in this recent mommy race among the stars (Almond 1998).

'Intensive mothering' and the 'new momism' are among some of the newest social and cultural trends. These cultural ideologies have been developing their values since the early 1990s. A 'new traditionalist' campaign was born in many women's magazines. *Good Housekeeping* and *Vogue*, among others, started to portray this 'new momism' with great pressure to perform. The performance standards are actually even higher than for the 1950s stay-at-home 'blissful cake baker housewife'. Children are shown as cool accessories and motherhood as an idealised image of perfect women and families. By the late 1990s, a hyper-natalism emerged and it was named: 'the new sexy moms!' (Douglas and Meredith 2005). Many celebrities continue making magazine front covers, explaining that it is much more rewarding to raise children than to be a rich, A-list star. Mothers are discussed in sexualised language: 'yummy mummy', 'slummy mummy', 'hot mama'. A new maternal lexicon circulates in popular culture and is present in a multitude of forums in the internet. Terms include mompreneur (entrepreneur), momager (manager), momoirist (memoir writer), celebmom (celebrity), momzilla (controlling), martyr mommy (overly, self-sacrificial) and sanctimommy (sanctimonious). Acronyms include SMUMs (smart, middle-class, uninvolved mothers), SAHMs (stay-at-home moms) and SCAMS (smart, child-centred, active moms).

A recent, and perhaps the most influential, study of mothers in contemporary popular culture is: *The Mommy Myth: The Idealizations of Motherhood and How it has Undermined All Women* (Douglas and Meredith 2005). This book introduces the 'new momism' as a variation on Hays's 'intensive mothering' (Hays 1998b). Thus, the two terms can be used interchangeably, as they refer to the same cultural/social ideology in relation to maternity. It is possible to argue that what the 'feminine mystique' was in the 1960s, 'intensive mothering' was in the 1990s and the 'new momism' is in the twenty-first century.

Maternal ambivalence is the direct consequence of these cultural trends. 'Intensive mothering' separates love and hate and keeps the 'dark side of motherhood' in the unconscious. By not integrating these two polarities in the experience of motherhood, a masochistic self-denial emerges in the mother's psyche (Hays 1998). Adrienne Rich exemplified this struggle when she wrote:

> My children cause me the most exquisite suffering of which I have any experience ... these tiny beings, monsters of selfishness and intolerance. There are times when I feel only death will free us from one another, when I envy the barren women who has the luxury of her regrets but lives a life of

privacy and freedom. I love them. But it's in the enormity and inevitability of this love that the sufferings lie.

(1976, 1)

The 'exquisite suffering' that Rich writes about is the complex maternal relationship that is often denied in the cultural and social narratives of the twenty-first century. The consequences of this denial at a societal level are devastating. Research has shown how guilt, stress and depression are often the most common feelings that mothers encounter (Walls 2007). Maternal guilt has been found to take place in all cultures, races and economic statuses (Borisoff 2005). It is the aversive feeling that the person is doing something wrong and violating moral principles (Klass 1988). When cultural expectations, reinforced by the social network of communities, are in conflict with the authentic experience that mothers feel, the perceived maternal role must be in question.

Women do most of the caring of children. The ethics of care, and the importance that women place on relational interactions creates a responsibility for the wellbeing of others (Elvin-Nowak 1999). This responsibility is a double-edged sword, as it becomes the source of conflicting choices that consequently often produce the feelings of guilt (Gilligan 1982). It is understandable how these conflicting choices would enhance stress in the maternal space. Those who become mothers undergo a 'loss of identity' that is not only cultural but social, professional, somatic, spiritual and cognitive. These changes are further complicated by the extensive needs and demands of children (Thompson 1996). Mothers often choose to deny the so called 'negative' aspects of motherhood, and so mourn loss and grieve in isolation. The cultural context can collude to ostracise the individual who exposes the denial from which the cultural system operates (Parks 1998; Johnston and Swanson 2003).

Foucault (1977, 109) writes about this double bind dilemma as: 'The situation that women face where hegemonic power is preserved by the construction of ideals that can be successfully fulfilled by the dominant group but ensures the failure of subordinate groups'. For mothers, the biggest sphere in which this cultural ideology operates is in the dichotomy of the question of whether to stay at home or go out to work for pay. In this question, mothers will face the real 'hegemonic power' of the economy and the marketplace.

Motherhood and employment

Intense cultural conceptualisations of motherhood often polarise women. As indicated, the term 'mommy wars' was coined to define the dichotomy between stay-at-home mothers and working mothers. The terms 'working mothers', referring to paid working mothers, and 'full time mothers', referring to stay-at-home mothers, are obsolete. All mothers are working mothers and all mothers are full-time mothers. The media has been complicit in these wars by not accurately representing the forces at play for mothers who do and do not work outside the home (O'Reilly 2010).

Culturally, this polarisation is more marked in developed countries, and upper middle-class circles therein, where women usually have the 'economic choice' to stay at home. It is paramount to note that choices are manipulated to serve the economy and the market place of industrialised, developed countries. This arises from the way the institution of motherhood is marketed. The niche marketing of all stages of motherhood is targeted at all social economic classes. Mothers are encouraged to look 'hot' after birth and buy all types of brand accessories for themselves and for their babies. Research has shown that women use well-dressed and groomed children to confirm identities as 'good mothers', and to protect and enhance their own self-concepts during the course of everyday social interaction (Collett 2005).

These cultural trends serve the economy in such a way that it becomes very difficult to 'juggle' family and work and serve the imperatives of intensive mothering. Prevailing ideologies also reinforce the separation between the maternal space and the workplace. Families do not often have open and flexible work schedules supported by legislation. The relationship of gender, power and the economy construct a system in which mothers are at a clear disadvantage.

The work–life balance, although a European Union policy priority, varies considerably between different countries. The Nordic welfare states offer the highest level of support. It is important to note that the level of women's employment in individual nation states are not only a reflection of state family supports for caring, but also of wider economic, labour market policies such as tax systems, employment protections and regulations. Thus, the UK and US have the highest levels of employment amongst women, but not the highest family supports system for employed parents. The Nordic countries (Finland, Norway, Sweden and Denmark) have the more generous dual-earner family supports to be found in Europe (Gornick and Meyers 2003). Second-wave feminism has a big influence on policy in Scandinavian countries. This change has contributed to the process of 'feminising social citizenship' (Anttonen 2002) in those countries creating provisions for dual-earner family support and childcare, making a positive contribution to women's equality. These policies came with the change in the gender structures within Nordic societies. State supports for families are accompanied by the encouragement of men to undertake a greater share of domestic work and childcare. The Nordic states make a good provision for public day-care services, as well as paid parental leave and caring entitlements (Crompton and Lyonette 2006).

The reality is that European Union members face a great challenge to integrate women into the individualised worker model after the Lisbon European Council (2010). In this council, goals such as embracing a 'European social model', by building 'an active welfare state', were discussed. Work and family reconciliation have been on the agenda of social policies in the European community since the 1957 Treaty of Rome. These goals are built on a model of 'adult worker identity'. European governments are committed to achieving this model of independence and self-sufficiency for all individuals in the labour market (Coakley 2005) as well as ensuring higher female labour market participation.

Unequal gender divisions of labour in the family, work/family commitment reconciliation and gender equality in the workplace are still very fraught issues. Stay-at-home mothers can be highly valued but on the other hand, mothers are under pressure to be employed full time (Daly 2004). This dichotomous pattern is the same across European countries (Dean 2001; Dex 2003; Reynolds and Healy 2008). I conducted a survey in Dublin, Ireland (2014) with 100 mothers, and the results elucidated some of these issues concerning how mothers integrate the choices of 'being there for their children' and 'being a citizen worker' (Molina 2014).

Mothers hold the ambivalence between the two spheres (the private and the public) and the cultural and the social are the main constructions that facilitate this perpetuating process.

It is true that the cultural picture is changing as, increasingly, mothers have claimed a 'cybervoice' over the last decade. The first 'mommy blog' was written in 2005. The majority of these narratives document a realistic picture of personal, maternal reflections on maternal identity and ambivalence. As we leave the industrialised world for the technological world, it is worth noting that new technologies are making mothers freer to talk in a globalised forum. In 2006, the inaugural BlogHer conference about women bloggers made a statement on how mommy blogging is a radical act to change the institution of motherhood. This 'mamasphere' contains a great range of political opinions, debates on legislation affecting mothers and families, activism and personal maternal experiences (Kennedy 2007). This new cyberspace may be considered as the newest feminist frontier for mothers (Ross and Byerly 2004). This new technological tool is giving mothers a powerful voice. Research and assessment of the evolution of this medium in motherhood construction is in its infancy.

The social and cultural constructions of motherhood are probably the largest system within which the institution of motherhood operates. Educating women on how this influence of socially-constructed motherhood is oppressive is crucial for women's health and identity. Women lose their personal identities in this monopolisation of motherhood, which steals time, creates illusions and displaces their sense of meaning and purpose from their inner self to their children, and their role as mothers. This is perhaps one of the biggest challenges that women need to face in their own psychological, economic, social and spiritual development as human beings. The capacity to integrate the dichotomies in motherhood is crucial in this process. Developing the capacity to love – not the unrealistic ideal maternal love that culture advocates, but the love that encompasses the light and the dark moments – is an opportunity for thought, compromise and growth (Almond 1998).

Psychological dimensions of motherhood

The majority of psychological theories are child centred and are concentrated on the role of mothers in the development of the infant. Psychoanalytic, object relations, attachment theory as well as social and developmental psychology, are among the theoretical frameworks in which motherhood has been conceptualised over the past 100 years. This section focuses mainly on psychoanalytic psychology. Psychoanalysis has both theoretical and clinical applications and its intersection ranges from feminism, psychotherapy and sociology to art and popular culture. Chronologically, the birth of psychoanalysis came about with the discourse of 'hysteria', in 1890. Hysteria, as an 'illness', challenged the medical community because it had no organic cause. Hysteria demonstrated that there was more to illness than the organic body, which, in turn, contributed to all of Freud's psychoanalytic classical theories of the unconscious, sexuality and gendered complexes. By the end of the 1930s, there was another shift in psychoanalytic theory with the writings of Melanie Klein, Donald Winnicott and object relation theorists. Second-wave feminism followed with another change in psychoanalytic theory by challenging, critiquing and often rejecting some of the classical Freudian theories. Later, by 1968, the French feminists emerged (Luce Irigaray, Julia Kristeva and Helene Cixous) and a 'return' to psychoanalysis occurred through Lacanian thoughts. By the 1980s and 1990s, psychoanalytic feminism turned to the sociology of gender, and theorists such as Nancy Chodorow picked up where Winnicott left off, by considering the social context of the mother and the gendered ramifications of early maternal care. Currently, the postmodern turn has brought emphasis onto the subjective experience of motherhood – thoughts, feelings, wishes, desires and inner conflicts experienced through mothering. Maternal subjectivity is the recent psychoanalytic feminist theorising influenced by postmodern deconstructions of identity, intrapsychic phenomena and the social and cultural realms.

Psychoanalysis and mothering is a deep and complex theory and to have an extensive discussion will take many pages. In the following sections, a brief review of some of the psychoanalytic theories in relation to the maternal is outlined. The first section concentrates on the evolution from Freud to Lacan, and later to the post-Lacanian French feminists and their view on maternal subjectivity – a concept that is continuously studied in the current postmodern context. The object relation and attachment theories are also discussed as they offer a unique contribution that follows to some of the latest mothering practices (i.e. intensive mothering and the new momism) of our time. The final section discussed maternal ambivalence as the experience that is at the core of maternal, psychological development in our society.

Psychoanalysis and motherhood

Classic psychoanalysis is interested in motherhood through child development. Freud viewed motherhood as a stage in women's ego development and stated that unresolved issues and anxieties will surface in motherhood. He considered motherhood as part of a woman's psychosexual development, significant in the establishment of adult identity (Freud 1914).[4] Problems such as infertility or depression were seen in psychoanalysis as evidence of a woman's poor adjustment to adult female identity (Benjamin 1988).

In this classic theory of psychoanalysis, the central focus is on the father. The Oedipus complex is placed at the core of the human psyche and denotes the emotions and ideas that the mind keeps in the unconscious, via dynamic repression, that concentrates upon a child's desire to sexually possess the parent of the opposite sex (males attracted to their mothers, whereas females are attracted to their fathers). Lacan later reinforced this complex by portraying the mother as a devouring, controlling force from which the child must detach itself (Lacan 1985). This conceptualisation of the loss of the mother's subjectivity creates many difficulties in the daughter-mother relationship.

French feminists such as Kristeva and Irigaray have, however, developed theories in which women's biology and experience are included. They maintained that the classic psychoanalytic theory is phallic-centred, disempowering and oppressive to motherhood.

Kristeva questioned this psychoanalytic theory of the necessity of the violent maternal separation. For her, maternity co-exists on the border between the social and the biological. She believes the mother represents the nature/culture threshold, the limits to language, the point at which biology is instilled into 'the very body of a symbolizing subject' (Kristeva 1975). The maternal body is the place in which the splitting occurs and as a consequence, maternal identity is always under threat, divided and in process (Kristeva 1975). Kristeva sees the maternal neither as a subject[5] nor an object,[6] but 'the materialization of the split subject', the subject that is both same and other[7] (Kristeva 1975).

The 'symbolic' arises through the repression of the 'semiotic'. This semiotic is the phase prior to culture and language shaping the maternal form of signification. This signification opened and shifted to the pregnant body and at mothering, yielded the model of human relations, constantly negotiating. The signification is an inter-subjectivity, the capacity for mutual recognition for both mother-subject and child-subject to coexist (Benjamin 1988). Kristeva's aim was for the mother to realise that the birth of a child constitutes access to the 'other'. The mother experiences her being as a being for an 'other'. Therefore, mothers will not look for the phallus but instead understand that the 'true other' is within her (Oliver 1998). This theory challenged directly the concept of Freudian 'penis envy'.

Irigaray (1985b, 233) also claims that a woman's 'indefinite, in-finite, form is never complete in her ... but she is becoming that expansion that she neither is nor will be at any moment as definable universe'. She extends this notion to motherhood as the tension between the woman and mother with the singularity of the child:

> And for her, the danger of motherhood is that of it/her being arrested in the world of one child. If she closes up around the unit(y) of that conception, enfolds herself around that one, her desire will harden. Will become phallic because of this relation to the one?
>
> (Irigaray 1985b, 229)

The transition to motherhood is a certain disintegration – being a 'subject-in-process/on trial' (Kristeva 1974/1984, 101), as Kristeva termed it. There is a creative potential in this state and Irigaray uses the motion of transformation to figure the feminine itself. She believes that the key to maternal transformation is the release of the creative potential of restrictive practices and discourses through engagement rather than critique (Baraitser 2009).

Psychoanalytic theory has presented a unique challenge for social and cultural critique since its birth. The core of how women care for themselves and for others, is the fundamental question in motherhood, and continues to be the focus of psychoanalytic studies. Psychoanalysis continues to contribute greatly to the profound understanding of the gendered implications to care and the inter-subjectivity of the 'maternal space' in a capitalist and consumerist society.

Object relations and motherhood

During the 1940s, object relations theory contested the classical psychoanalytical view of the role of the mother. This model gave more significant importance to the mother and how she shapes the baby's experience. There is a notable theoretical shift in making the mother more visible, but on the other hand, an idealised and objectified maternal figure also emerged in the new framework. The 'good enough mother' concept, developed by Donald Winnicott, is characterised by the conditions that the mother needs to provide for the development of the child's concept of self (Winnicott 1957).

Professor Nancy Chodorow has further developed object relations theory, as well as the social construction of gender formation and identity, and consequently the psychology of motherhood. Her groundbreaking book, *The Reproduction of Mothering*, is a classic and one of the most influential books in the field of sociology and psychoanalysis (Chodorow 1978). One of her tasks was to explain and challenge how scientific theory accounted for women's desire for motherhood and for female centrality in childcare across cultures and historical eras. She determined that the cultural belief that childrearing is the woman's responsibility became the main foundation for male dominance and for political oppression of women. She contested (1978, 39) that: 'Women's capacities for mothering and abilities to get gratification from motherhood is strongly internalised, as well as psychologically and culturally enforced, and are built developmentally into the feminine psychic structure'. She also challenged prevailing perspectives on the mother–child relationship and how this relationship differed, depending on the child's gender. Using object relation theory, she asserted that mothers feel a stronger sense of unity with daughters because they share the same sex while they feel a sense of 'other' with sons, despite the closeness of the maternal bond. She asserted that these object relations also depend on the mothers' perception of these relationships, both on the conscious and unconscious levels (Chodorow 1978). These frameworks directly challenge the classic understanding of the Oedipal complex.

Another important contribution of her work pertains to the family's role in shaping the individual gender identity that reinforces social and cultural gender roles. Her theories open an important societal discourse in relation to motherhood, with the main question arising being: what is the result of being parented by a woman?

Women are the main parent and the main caregiver across cultures. Because women care for children, heterosexual symbiosis then has a different 'meaning' for men and women. Only in the last decade has research grown in awareness of the importance of the roles of fathers. Historically, there has been a pattern of excluding fathers from research of clinical/paediatric issues (Silverstein 2002). Nevertheless, fathers have been found to influence every characteristic studied in child development (Tamis-LeMonda and Cabrera 2014).

Women's sole responsibility for parenting, on a daily basis in society, is one of the core reasons that the institution of motherhood and families create gendered children. A profound challenge to the understanding of the engendering of motherhood is needed in order to break this cycle.

Attachment theory

Attachment theory as developed by John Bowlby investigated motherhood through the process of establishing a secure bond between the mother and child. Without this secure attachment, the child's social and emotional development is in danger. Bowlby's research embraced new understanding in the fields of evolutionary biology, aetiology, developmental psychology and cognitive science. He proposed that there are mechanisms underlying an infant's emotional link with the caregiver(s) as a result of evolutionary pressure (Cassidy 1999).

The biggest development in attachment theory in relation to motherhood is the ideology of attachment parenting. This term was coined by paediatrician William Sears, in his famous book *The Attachment Parenting Book*. This philosophy asserts that attachment parenting and the child's formation of a secure attachment construct, is vital to the child's survival and for the parents to meet most children's needs promptly. Also, children become capable of communicating their needs to adults within this process (Sears 2001).

There has been heavy criticism of developments in attachment theory. Feminist researchers believe that intensive mothering is the direct consequence, in our society, of the influence of attachment theories and their propagation. Women have found attachment parenting strenuous and demanding, and they place the blame for this kind of cultural philosophy on a social commitment to a 'culture of total motherhood', which in turn leads to an 'age of anxiety and perfectionism in motherhood' (Warner 2006). Sociologist Sharon Hays argues that this ideology of intensive mothering by attachment parenting makes parents, and especially mothers, totally responsible for unrealistic obligations, and perpetuates a 'double shift' life for working women (Hays 1998b). The maternal image of attachment theory has been challenged and has yielded to a much more subjective and complex one. Studies on maternal ambivalence paint a picture that is very different from the 'good enough' mother.

Unravelling maternal ambivalence

As discussed above, the idealisation of motherhood (through strong cultural and normative social messages) reinforces and hides the experience of maternal ambivalence. Research through qualitative sociological studies has suggested that ambivalence is a multidimensional phenomenon with distinct presentations and pathways associated within different social groups (Connidis and McMullin 2002; Fong and Larissa 2002; Leibovich 2006; Wilson *et al.* 2006). The 'illusory mask' (Maushart 1999) that disguises the true reality of the motherhood experience represents one of the core factors in maternal ambivalence (Lupton 2000).

Ambivalence is defined as having both psychologically conflicting feelings, cognitions and motivations at a subjective level, which arise from a contradiction of the social norm of the social-structural level (O'Reilly 2010). Ambivalence is a combination of the feelings of love and hatred we experience towards those who are important to us. Psychologically, it is a normal phenomenon. The problem arises when such a phenomenon is shamed, demonised and hidden from cultural discourse.

Fictional writers have examined this theme in very important literature, including *Rosemary's Baby* (Levin 1967), *Beloved* (Morrison 1987), *The Fifth Child* (Lessing 1988) and *We Need to Talk about Kevin* (Shriver 2003). Even Shelley's *Frankenstein* (1823) hinted at women's fears of monstrous births (Almond 1998). Virginia Woolf's *To the Lighthouse* (Woolf 1927) is an example of the maternal ideal as a pre-Raphaelite Madonna who is benevolent, delicate and eternal (Parker 2005).

In art, the mother–child relationship is a signifier of states of merging and of the complete and total unity of 'love'. This state has been described as the 'idealisation of primary narcissism' (Kristeva 1986, 161). Similarly, Erikson describes religion as 'the simple and fervent wish for a hallucinatory sense of unity with the maternal matrix' (1968, 263). And romantic love has also been related to the dynamics of the longing for infantile bliss and plenitude within the mother–child fusion (Person 2006). The perceived bonding of mother and child sets cultural expectations that the mother must be completely fulfilled by such a relationship. Archetypically, these powerful and profound belief systems are embedded in our society. Thus, the denial of ambivalence is present in mothers' collective psyche, almost by osmosis.

British psychoanalyst Joan Raphael-Leff has written extensively about the internal world of mothers (1991; 2001; 2003). She claims that motherhood may be a process that leads to a resolution of childhood conflicts. Infants force into awareness split-off aspects of the parents' self, producing a re-experiencing of helplessness, neediness, frustration and abandonment (Baraitser 2009). The mother has to 'bear' the subjective unconscious feelings such as hatred, ambivalence, failure, shame and guilt. To tolerate these feelings of 'suffering', often unaided by the cultural context, creates a very confusing matrix for mothers, who do so at an intrapsychic level. Very little research has been carried out about the way the mother struggles to transform these processes at a spiritual level.

Conclusions

Culturally and psychologically, the mother is represented as the vehicle and the facilitator to the developing child. A parallel dynamic process is in operation in maternal ambivalence that is well worth paying attention to. There is spiritually transformative and creative potential in maternal ambivalence. It is a unique time when mothers can encounter themselves unconsciously through an encounter with the child (Baraitser 2009).

Psychotherapist Rozsika Parker (2005) agrees with Raphael-Leff in the belief that maternal ambivalence is the core for maternal psychological development. Unmanageable ambivalence develops into anxiety, depression and a wide range of feelings from guilt to shame. Awareness nurtured through intentional attentiveness is one of the main capacities that will help the mother to achieve a full and profound understanding of her intrapsychic processes in relation to her own self-autonomy and her responsibility towards the baby. This creative transformation may happen at various levels.

It has been observed, clinically, that, by becoming aware and conscious of these maternal ambivalent feelings, women can create new initiatives and resources for themselves and for their children (Christie and Correia 1987). Making connections with these deep, inner spiritual resources enhances the capacity, power and the authority to mother. Awareness practices also promote consciousness and understanding that maternal ambivalence is not a problem – rather, the challenge is how the mother manages the guilt and anxiety that it provokes (Parker 2005). The struggle becomes much more complicated when the tension between the psychical and social mother is accentuated by the cultural and social influences of the institution of motherhood (Parker 2005).

It is crucial to figure out how the awareness, development, understanding and application of spiritual practices may contribute to resolving such ambivalence. How spiritual capacities can assist mothers is paramount to understanding the role of spirituality in the transition to empowered motherhood.

In the next chapter, the turn to spirituality in our contemporary society is mapped. Contemporary spirituality is understood very differently from previous centuries. The analysis of intrinsic human spiritual capacities may contribute to the complex transformation that may empower the mother from within.

Thus, the investigation of the emergence of maternal, spiritual capacities in the transition to motherhood is a valuable contribution to the current inner empowerment discussion. How spiritual capacities can assist mothers is crucial to understanding the role of spirituality in the transition to empowered motherhood.

Notes

1 The term 'Republican Motherhood' was first coined in the late 1970s by American historian Linda Kerber (1980), while examining Mary Wollstonecraft's publication: *A Vindication of the Rights of Woman*.
2 Lacan's original seminar was published in French as 'Le Seminaire, Livre XX, ENCORE, 1972–1973', by Editions du Seuil, Paris, 1975.
3 Excerpt from my own conference notes.
4 Sigmund Freud, in his famous 1914 essay 'On Narcissism', indicated that because a daughter cannot clearly distinguish herself from her mother, no clear sense of self develops in women. Without a clear sense of self, women never fully develop into mature, moral beings.
5 In psychoanalysis, the 'subject' is not the Cartesian vision of a centred and autonomous 'I'. The subject's autonomy and self-awareness is constantly undermined by impulses from the Id and by the pressures of the Superego. A good way to understand the differences between theoretical approaches is to examine what they emphasise in (and leave out of) their accounts of the human subject. Feminism, for example, may pay particular attention to the body as a site of cultural impositions based on gender norms.
6 In psychoanalysis, the 'object', the passive thing that serves as the content of conscious observation, is contrasted with the 'subject', the conscious agent who observes the object. Psychoanalysis describes 'objects' that are invested with libidinal energy. These 'objects' can be other people (the 'object of one's affections') or anything else (including abstract concepts like 'of freedom' or 'justice') that serves as a focal point desire.
7 In psychoanalysis, the mirror stage of psychosexual development creates an image of the ego as an ideal I for the subject. This Ideal-I becomes an 'other' within the subject's experience of his or her 'I', a component of a 'self' that is internally divided.

References

Abrams, L. 2002. *The Making of a Modern Woman*. Upper Saddle River, USA: Pearson.

Allen, A. 2005. *Feminism and Motherhood in Western Europe*. New York: Palgrave Macmillan.

Allen, J. 1986. *Motherhood: The Annihilation of Women. Lesbian Philosophy: Explorations*. Palo Alto, USA: Institute of Lesbian Studies.

Almond, B. 1998. 'The Monster Within: Mary Shelley's Frankenstein and a Patient's Fears of Childbirth and Mothering'. *International Journal of Psychoanalysis* 75:775–786.

Anttonen, A. 2002. 'Universalism and Social Policy: A Nordic-Feminist Revaluation'. *Nora Nordic Journal of Women's Studies* 10(2):71–80.

Apple, R. 2006. *Perfect Motherhood; Science and Childrearing in America*. New Brunswick, USA: Rutgers University Press.

Armstrong, K. 2001. *The Battle for God: Fundamentalism in Judaism, Christianity and Islam*. London: HarperCollins Publishers.

Atkinson, C. 1991. *The Oldest Vocation: Christian Motherhood in the Middle Ages*. Ithaca, USA: Cornell University Press.

Aughterson, K. ed. 1995. *Renaissance Woman; A Sourcebook: Constructions of Femininity in England*. New York: Routledge.

Baraitser, L. 2009. *Maternal Encounters. The Ethics of Interruption. Women and Psychology*. London: Routledge.

Baumgardner, J. 2011. *F'em! Goo Goo, Gaga, and Some Thoughts on Balls*. Berkeley, USA: Seal Press.

Benjamin, J. 1988. *The Bonds of Love: Psychoanalysis, Feminism and the Problem of Domination*. New York: Pantheon.

Borisoff, D. 2005. 'Transforming Motherhood: We've Come a Long Way, Maybe'. *Review of Communication* 5:1–11.

Boyer, J. 2000. *Enduring Voices: Document Sets to Accompany the Enduring Vision. A History of the American People: The Cult of Domesticity and the Reaction: From True Women to New Women*. Lexington, USA: D.C. Heath.

Bradley, K. 1991. *Discovering the Roman Family*. London: Oxford University Press.

Brown, S., Lumley, J., Small, R., and Astbury, J. 1994. *Missing Voices: The Experience of Motherhood*. Melbourne: Oxford University Press.

Burke, P., and Kwan, D. 1993. *Family Values: Two Moms and Their Son*. New York: Random House Inc.

Butler, J. 2000. 'Longing for Recognition: Commentary on the Work of Jessica Benjamin. Roundtable on the Work of Jessica Benjamin'. *Studies in Gender and Sexuality* 1(3):271–290.

Cantarella, E. 1987. *Pandora's Daughters: The Role and Status of Women in Greek and Roman Antiquity*. Baltimore, USA: Johns Hopkins University Press.

Cassidy, J. 1999. 'The Nature of a Child's Ties'. In *Handbook of Attachment: Theory, Research and Clinical Applications*, edited by J. Cassidy and P. R. Shaver, 3–20. New York: Guilford Press.

Chandler, M. 1998. 'Emancipated Subjectivities and the Subjugation of Mothering Practices'. In *Redefining Motherhood: Changing Identities and Patterns*, edited by S. Abbey and A. O'Reilly, 270–286. Toronto: Second Story Press.

Chodorow, N. 1978. *The Reproduction of Mothering: Psychoanalysis and the Sociology of Gender*. Berkeley, USA: University of California Press.

Choi, P., Henshaw, C., Baker, S., and Tree, J. 2005. 'Supermum, Superwife, Supereverything: Performing Femininity in the Transition to Motherhood'. *Journal of Reproductive and Infant Psychology* 23:167–180.

Christie, G., and Correia, A. 1987. 'Maternal Ambivalence in a Group Analytic Setting'. *British Journal of Psychotherapy* 3(3):205–215.

Cixous, H. 1975. 'Breaths'. In *The Helene Cixous Reader*, edited by S. Sellers, 47–57. London: Routledge.

Coakley, A. 2005. *Mothers, Welfare and Labour Market Activation*. Dublin: Combat Poverty Agency.

Cobb, M. 2012. 'An Amazing 10 Years: The Discovery of Egg and Sperm in the 17th Century'. *Reproduction in Domestic Animals* 47(4):2–6.

Collett, J. 2005. 'What Kind of Mother Am I? Impression Management and the Social Construction of Motherhood'. *Symbolic Interaction* 28(3):327–347.

Connidis, I., and McMullin, J. 2002. 'Sociological Ambivalence and Family Ties: A Critical Perspective'. *Journal of Marriage and Family* 64:558–567.

Crawford, B. 2011. 'Third-Wave Feminism, Motherhood and the Future of Feminist Legal Theory'. In *Gender, Sexualities and Law*, edited by J. Jones, A. Grear, A. Fenton, and K. Stevenson, 227–240. New York: Routledge.

Crittenden, A. 2001. *The Price of Motherhood: Why the Most Important Job in the World is Still the Least Valued*. New York: Henry Holt.

Crompton, R., and Lyonette, C. 2006. 'Work–Life "Balance" in Europe'. *Acta Sociologica* 49(4):379–393.

Dally, A. 1983. *Inventing Motherhood: The Consequences of an Ideal*. New York: Schocken Books.

Daly, M. 2004. 'Families, and Family Life in Ireland: Challenges for the Future'. *Report of Public Consultation Fora*. Dublin: Department of Social and Family Affairs.

Darnton, N. 1990. 'Mommy Vs. Mommy'. *Newsweek*. www.newsweek.com/mommy-vs-mommy-206132.

De Beauvoir, S. 1949. *The Second Sex*. London: Vintage.

Dean, H. 2001. 'Working Parenthood and Parental Obligation'. *Critical Social Policy* 21:3.

Dex, S. 2003. *Families and Work in the Twenty-first Century*. York, UK: Policy Press.

Dinnerstein, D. 1976. *The Mermaid and the Minotaur: Sexual Arrangements and Human Malaise*. Michigan, USA: Harper and Row.

Douglas, S., and Meredith, M. 2005. *The Mommy Myth: The Idealization of Motherhood and How it Has Undermined All Women*. Florence, USA: Free Press Publishers.

Downing, C. 1994. *The Long Journey Home. Revisioning the Myth of Demeter and Persephone for Our Time*. Boulder, USA: Shambhala Publications.

Elvin-Nowak, Y. 1999. 'The Meaning of Guilt: A Phenomenological Description of Employed Mother's Experiences of Guilt'. *Scandinavian Journal of Psychology* 40:73–83.

Ennis, L. ed. 2014. *Intensive Mothering: The Cultural Contradictions of Modern Motherhood*. Bradford, Canada: Demeter Press.

Epstein, R. 2010. *Get Me Out. A History of Childbirth from the Garden of Eden to the Sperm Bank*. New York: W. W. Norton & Company.

Erdrich, L. 1995. *The Blue Jay's Dance: A Birth Year*. New York: HarperCollins Publishing.

Erikson, E. 1968. *Young Man Luther*. New York: Norton.

Firestone, S. 1970. *The Dialectic of Sex: The Case for Feminist Revolution*. New York: William Morrow and Company.

Fong, C., and Larissa, Z. 2002. 'Dueling Experiences and Dual Ambivalences: Emotional and Motivational Ambivalence of Women in High Status Positions'. *Motivation and Emotion* 26(1):105–121.

Ford, L. 2008. *Encyclopedia of Women and American Politics*. New York: Facts on File.

Foucault, M. 1977. *Power/Knowledge. Selected Interviews and Other Writings 1972–1977*. New York: Pantheon Books.

Freud, S. 1914. *Zur Einführung des Narzißmus (On Narcisism)*. Vienna: Internationaler Psychoanalytischer Verlag.

Friedan, B. 1963. *The Feminine Mystique*. New York: Norton.

Fuller, Margaret. 1845. *Woman in the Nineteenth Century*. Cambridge, USA: Greeley & McElrath.

Gies, F., and Gies, J. 1987. *Marriage and the Family in the Middle Ages*. New York: Harper & Row.

Gilligan, C. 1982. *In a Different Voice*. Boston, USA: Harvard University Press.

Gillis, S., Howie, G., and Munford, R. eds 2007. *Third Wave Feminism: A Critical Exploration*. London: Palgrave Macmillan.

Gornick, J., and Meyers, M. 2003. *Families that Work*. New York: Russell Sage Foundation.

Grayzel, S. 2002. *Women and the First World War. Seminar Studies in History*. New York: Routledge.

Green, M. 2001. *The Trotula: A Medieval Compendium of Women's Medicine*. Philadelphia, USA: University of Pennsylvania Press.

Green, F. 2004. 'Feminist Mothers: Successfully Negotiating the Tensions between Motherhood as Institution and Experience'. In *Mother Outlaws: Theories and Practices of Empowered Mothering*, edited by A. O'Reilly, 31–43. Toronto: Canadian Scholars' Press.

Hays, S. 1998a. 'The Fallacious Assumptions and Unrealistic Prescriptions of Attachment Theory: A Comment on "Parents' Socioemotional Investment in Children"'. *Journal of Marriage and Family* 60(3):782–790.

Hays, S. 1998b. *The Cultural Contradictions of Motherhood*. New Haven, USA: Yale University Press.

Hewett, H. 2006. 'Talkin' bout a Revolution. Building a Mothers' Movement in the Third Wave'. *Journal of the Association for Research on Mothering* 8(1–2):34–53.

Horowitz, D. 1998. *Betty Friedan and the Making of the Feminine Mystique*. Amherst, USA: University of Massachusetts Press.

Horowitz, E. 2004. 'Resistance as a Site of Empowerment: The Journey away from Maternal Sacrifice'. In *Mother Outlaws: Theories and Practices of Empowered Mothering*, edited by A. O'Reilly, 43–58. Toronto: Canadian Scholars' Press.

Irigaray, L. 1985a. *This Sex Which is Not One*. Ithaca, USA: Cornell University Press.

Irigaray, L. 1985b. *Speculum of the Other Woman*, translated by G. C. Gill. Ithaca, USA: Cornell University Press.

Jackson, M. 1992. *The Mother Zone: Love, Sex, and Laundry in the Modern Family*. New York: Henry Holt & Co.

Jeremiah, E. 2002. 'Troublesome Practices: Mothering, Literature and Ethics'. *Journal of the Association for Research on Mothering* 4(2):7–16.

Jeremiah, E. 2006. 'Motherhood to Mothering and Beyond. Maternity in Recent Feminist Thought'. *Journal of the Association for Research on Mothering* 8(1/2):21–33.

Jetter, A., Anelise O., and Taylor, D. 1997. *The Politics of Motherhood: Activist Voices from Left to Right*. Lebanon, USA: University Press of New England.

Johnston, D., and Swanson, D. 2003. 'Undermining Mothers: A Content Analysis of the Representations of Mothers in Magazines'. *Mass Communication & Society* 6:262.

Kennedy, T. 2007. 'The Personal is Political: Feminist Blogging and Virtual Consciousness-Raising'. *The Scholar and Feminist Online* 5(2).

Kerber, L. 1980. *Women of the Republic: Intellect and Ideology in Revolutionary America*. Chapel Hill, USA: University of North Carolina Press.

Kimble, H. 2009. 'The Fourth Wave of Feminism: Psychoanalytic Perspectives Introductory Remarks'. *Studies in Gender and Sexuality* 10(4):185–189.

Kinser, A. 2010. *Motherhood and Feminism*. Jackson, USA: Seal Press.

Klass, E. 1988. 'Cognitive Behavioral Perspectives on Women and Guilt'. *Journal of Rational-Emotive and Cognitive-Behavior Therapy* 6:23–32.

Kristeva, J. 1974/1984. *Revolution in Poetic Language*, translated by M. Waller. New York: Columbia University Press.

Kristeva, J. 1975. *Desire in Language: A Semiotic Approach to Literature and Art*. New York: Columbia University Press.

Kristeva, J. 1986. 'Stabat Mater'. In *The Kristeva Reader*, edited by T. Moi. Oxford: Basil Blackwell.

Lacan, J. 1985. *Feminine Sexuality*. New York: Norton.

Lamott, A. 1994. *Operating Instructions: A Journal of My Son's First Year*. New York: Ballantine Books.

Lazarre, J. 1996. *Beyond the Whiteness of Whiteness: Memoir of a White Mother of Black Sons*. Durham, USA: Durham Duke University Press.

LeBeau, Claire. 2013. *Maternal Guilt: The Early Emotional Experiences of First-Time Mothers*. London: Scholars' Press.

Leibovich, L. 2006. *Maybe Baby: 28 Writers Tell the Truth about Skepticism, Infertility, Baby Lust, Childlessness, Ambivalence, and How They Made the Biggest Decision of Their Lives*. London: Harper Collins.

Lerner, G. 1993. *The Creation of Feminist Consciousness: From the Middles Ages to Eighteen-seventy*. New York: Oxford University Press.

Lessing, D. 1988. *The Fifth Child*. New York: Alfred A. Knopf.

Levin, I. 1967. *Rosemary's Baby*. New York: Random House.

Lindley, S.1996. *You Have Stept out of Your Place. A History of Women and Religion in America*. Westminster, UK: John Knox Press.

Linker, M. 2006. 'Explaining the World. Philosophical Reflections on Feminism and Mothering'. *Journal of the Association for Research on Mothering* 8(1/2):147–156.

Lupton, D. 2000. 'Love/Hate Relationships: The Ideals and Experiences of First-Time Mothers'. *Journal of Sociology* 36(1):50–63.

Maushart, S. 1999. *The Mask of Motherhood: How Becoming a Mother Changes Our Lives and Why We Never Talk about It*. Auckland, New Zealand: Penguin Books.

McDonnell, E. 2007. *Mama Rama: A Memoir of Sex, Kids & Rock 'n' Roll*. Cambridge, USA: Da Capo Press.

McDonough, C. 2006. 'Motherhood and Feminism. Lessons from the Titanic'. *Journal of the Association for Research on Mothering* 8(1/2):123–128.

McMahon, M. 1995. *Engendering Motherhood: Identity and Self-Transformation in Women's Lives*. New York: Guilford Press.

Middleton, A. 2006. 'Mothering under Duress. Examining the Inclusiveness of Feminist Mothering Theory'. *Journal of the Association for Research on Mothering* 8(1/2):72–82.

Miller, T. 2005. *Making Sense of Motherhood: A Narrative Approach*. Cambridge, UK: Cambridge University Press.

Millett, K. 1970. *Sexual Politics*. New York: Doubleday.

Mitchell, J. 1974. *Psychoanalysis and Feminism*. London: Virago.

Molina, N. 2014. 'Integrating Choices: "Being There for My Children" and "Being a Citizen Worker": Irish Survey on Stay-at-Home Mothers'. In *Stay-at-Home Mothers: Dialogues and Debates*, edited by E. Reid Boyd and G. Letherby, 139–153. Ontario, Canada: Demeter Press.

Morrison, T. 1987. *Beloved*. New York: Plume.

Munro, E. 2013. *Feminism: A Fourth Wave? Political Insight*. London: The Political Studies Association.

O'Brien, M. 1981. *The Politics of Reproduction*. Boston, USA: Routledge and Kegan Paul.

O'Reilly, A. 2004. *From Motherhood to Mothering: The Legacy of Adrienne Rich's Of Woman Born*. Albany, USA: SUNY Press.

O'Reilly, A. 2006. *Rocking the Cradle: Thoughts on Motherhood, Feminism and the Possibility of Empowered Mothering*. Toronto: Demeter Press.

O'Reilly, A. 2010. *Encyclopedia of Motherhood. Volume 2. Intensive Mothering*. London: Sage Publications.

O'Reilly, A. 2011. *The 21st Century Motherhood Movement: Mothers Speak Out on Why We Need to Change the World and How to Do It*. Toronto: Demeter Press.

Oliver, K. 1998. *Subjects without Subjectivity: From Abject Fathers to Desiring Mothers*. Lanham, USA: Rowan & Littlefield.

Orenstein, P. 2007. *Waiting for Daisy: A Tale of Two Continents, Three Religions, Five Infertility Doctors and Oscar, an Atomic Bomb, a Romantic Night and One Woman's Quest to Become a Mother.* New York: Bloomsbury.

Parker, R. 2005. *The Experience of Maternal Ambivalence. Torn in Two.* London: Virago Press.

Parks, C. 1998. 'Coping with Loss'. *British Medical Journal* 316:1521–1524.

Parton, N. 2008. 'The Social Construction of Reality: A Treatise in the Sociology of Knowledge, Peter L. Berger, and Thomas Luckman'. *Journal of Social Work* 38(4):823–824.

Patterson, M. 2008. *The American New Woman Revisited: A Reader, 1894–1930.* New Brunswick, USA: Rutgers University Press.

Person, E. 2006. *Dreams of Love and Fateful Encounters.* Arlington, VA: American Psychiatric Publishing.

Petrassi, D. 2012. ' "For Me, the Children Come First": A Discursive Psychological Analysis of How Mothers Construct Fathers' Roles in Childrearing and Childcare'. *Feminism & Psychology* 22:518–527.

Pocock, B. 2001. 'A Better Life Can Be Legislated'. *The Age* 5(9):14.

Pomeroy, S. 1991. *Women's History and Ancient History.* Chapel Hill, USA: University of North Carolina Press.

Raphael-Leff, J. 1991. *Psychological Processes of Childbearing.* London: Chapman & Hall.

Raphael-Leff, J. 2001. *Pregnancy – The Inside Story.* London: Karnac Publications.

Raphael-Leff, J., ed. 2003. *Parent-Infant Psychodynamics: Wild Things, Mirrors and Ghosts.* London: Whurr Publications.

Reynolds, B., and Healy, S. 2008. *Making Choices – Choosing Futures: Ireland at a Crossroads.* Dublin: CORI Justice.

Rich, A. 1976. *Of a Woman Born: Motherhood as Experience and Institution.* New York: W. W. Norton & Company, Inc.

Ross, A., and Purcell, B. 2004. *The Woman's Way to Wealth.* Dublin: Font Publications.

Ross, E. 1995. 'The Secret Lives of Mothers'. *Women's Review of Books* 7(6):6–7.

Ross, K., and Byerly, C. 2004. 'Cyberspace: The New Feminist Frontier?' In *Women and Media: International Perspectives*, edited by K. Ross and C. Byerly. Oxford, UK: Blackwell.

Rousseau, J. 2007. *Emile, or On Education.* Sioux Falls, USA: NuVision Publications.

Ruddick, S. 1989. *Maternal Thinking: Toward a Politics of Peace.* Boston, USA: Beacon Press.

Sears, W. 2001. *The Attachment Parenting Book: A Commonsense Guide to Understanding and Nurturing Your Baby.* Boston, USA: Little, Brown and Company.

Shelley, Mary. 1823. *Frankenstein.* London: G. and W. B. Whittaker.

Shriver, L. 2003. *We Need to Talk about Kevin.* New York: Perennial.

Silverstein, L. 2002. 'Fathers and Families'. In *Retrospect and Prospect in the Psychological Study of Families*, edited by J. McHale and W Groinick, 35–64. New York: Lawrence Eribaum Associates.

Smith, J. 2003. *A Potent Spell: Mother Love and the Power of Fear.* Boston, USA: Houghton Mifflin Harcourt.

Snow, D., and Anderson, L. 1987. 'Identity Work among the Homeless: The Verbal Construction and Avowal of Personal Identities'. *American Journal of Sociology* 92:1336–1371.

Sommerville, J. ed. 1991. *Filmer: Patriarcha and Other Writing.* Cambridge, UK: Cambridge University Press.

Sotirin, P. 2010. 'Autoethnographic Mother-Writing: Advocating Radical Specificity'. *Journal of Research Practice* 6(1):Article M9.

Stevens, H. 2008. *Henry James and Sexuality*. Cambridge, UK: Cambridge University Press.

Tamis-LeMonda, C .S., and Cabrera, N. eds 2014. *Handbook of Father Involvement: Multidisciplinary Perspectives*. London: Routledge.

Tardy, R. 2000. 'But I Am a Good Mom. The Social Construction of Motherhood through Healthcare Conversations'. *Journal of Contemporary Ethnography* 29:433–473.

Thompson, S. 1996. 'Barriers to Maintaining a Sense of Meaning and Control in the Face of Loss'. *Journal of Personal and Intrapersonal Loss* 1:333–357.

Tilly, L., and Scott, J. 1989. *Women, Work and Family*. New York: Routledge.

Turnbull, L. 2006. 'The Dilemmas of Feminist Activism in Law'. *Journal of the Association for Research on Mothering* 8(1/2):129–134.

Tyldesley, J. 1984. *Daughters of Isis: Women in Ancient Egypt*. New York: Penguin.

Walker, R. 2007. *Baby Love: Choosing Motherhood after a Lifetime of Ambivalence*. New York: Riverhead Books.

Walls, L. 2007. *The Social Construction of Motherhood: Implications and Interventions*. http://dtpr.lib.athabascau.ca/action/download.php?filename=caap/loriwallsfinalproject.pdf.

Warner, J. 2006. *Perfect Madness: Motherhood in the Age of Anxiety*. New York: Riverhead Books.

Waugh, P. 1989. 'Stalemates? Feminists, Postmodernists and Unfinished Issues'. In *Modern Aesthetics. Modern Literary Theory; A Reader*, edited by P. Rice and P. Waugh, 322–341. London: Arnold.

Wilson, A., Kim, M., Glen, H., and Wickrama, K. 2006. 'Ambivalence in Mother-Adult Child Relations: A Dyadic Analysis'. *Social Psychology Quarterly* 69(3):235–252.

Winnicott, D. 1957. *The Child and the Family*. London: Tavistock.

Wolf, N. 2003. *Misconceptions: Truth, Lies, and the Unexpected on the Journey to Motherhood*. New York: Anchor Publishers.

Woolf, V. 1927. *To the Lighthouse*. London: Grafton Books.

Part II
Contemporary spirituality

2 Spiritual awakening

The cultural shift

Western society has witnessed social, psychological and cultural developments that are impacting the way populations understand the conceptualisation of spirituality. Value systems are changing in relation to family and the way children are raised. Spirituality is shaped by psychological, cultural, historical and biological dimensions. It is therefore of great importance to uncover recent spiritual developments in society.

Spirituality and society

Many social scientists and anthropologists claim that a profound cultural shift is taking place in Western society. This shift is described in the literature as a move towards a postmaterial, postmetaphysical and postsecular society (Campbell 2007; Gibson 2009; Tarnas 2007). A world value survey, which conducted representative national surveys in almost 100 countries stated:

> Although the authority of the established churches continues to decline, during the past twenty years the public of post-industrial societies have become increasingly likely to spend time thinking about the meaning and purpose of life. Whether one views these concerns as religious depends on one's definition of religion, but it is clear that the materialistic secularism of industrial society is fading. There is a shift from institutionally fixed forms of dogmatic religion to individually flexible forms of spiritual religion.
>
> (Inglehart and Welzel 2005, 31)

These developments have in the last few decades, led to an emergence of research in the study of spiritual experience, and many scholars now believe that spirituality needs to be researched in a broad sense in the population (Hedlund-de Witt 2011).

Cultural shift

The largest cross-cultural longitudinal study of changes in cultural beliefs, values and worldviews is the World Values Survey. The project has been undertaken by a global network of social scientists who have surveyed the basic values and beliefs of the publics of almost 100 societies, on all six continents.[1]

The surveys have been designed to provide a comprehensive measurement of all major areas of human concern, from religion to politics, to economic and social life. Two themes dominate the data:

1   Traditional versus secular-rational: this theme reflects the contrast between societies in which religion is very important and those in which it is not.
2   Survival versus self-expression: this theme is linked with the transition from industrial society to postindustrial societies, which brings a polarisation between survival and self-expression values.

The second theme is most evident in the Western world, in which wealth is unprecedented and there is an increasing population that has grown up taking survival for granted. Values have consequently shifted from ensuring economic and physical security to an increased emphasis on subjective wellbeing and self-expression (Inglehart and Welzel 2005; 2010). In almost all industrial and postindustrial societies, values have also shifted from traditional towards secular-rational values, and from survival values towards self-expression values. These values give priority to environmental protection, tolerance of diversity (including cultural background and sexual orientation) and gender equality. This shift has also affected childrearing values. There is much more emphasis on imagination, tolerance and trust as important values to teach a child. Societies that ranked high in self-expression values also tended to rank high in interpersonal trust. This postmaterial culture generally promotes freedom and self-expression and tends to have activist political orientations (Inglehart and Welzel 2010).

The World Value Survey Cultural Map (Figure 2.1) helpfully reflects the cultural proximity of different countries, as opposed to their geographical proximity. This proximity is measured according to their people's values. Traditional values emphasise the importance of religion, parent-child ties, deference to authority and traditional family values. People who embrace these values also reject divorce, abortion, euthanasia and suicide. These societies have high levels of national pride and a nationalistic outlook. Secular-rational values have the opposite preferences to the traditional values. These societies place less emphasis on religion, traditional family values and authority. Divorce, abortion, euthanasia and suicide are seen as relatively acceptable. (Suicide is not necessarily more common.) Survival values place emphasis on economic and physical security. They are linked with a relatively ethnocentric outlook and low levels of trust and tolerance. Self-expression values give high priority to environmental protection, growing tolerance of foreigners, gays and lesbians and gender equality and rising demands for participation in decision-making in economic and political life.

Because these major cultural changes are occurring, they point to a process of intergenerational value change, whereby the younger postmaterialist birth cohorts emphasise autonomy, self-expression and the quality of life. The study (Inglehart and Welzel 2008, 130) asserted that: 'We interpret contemporary

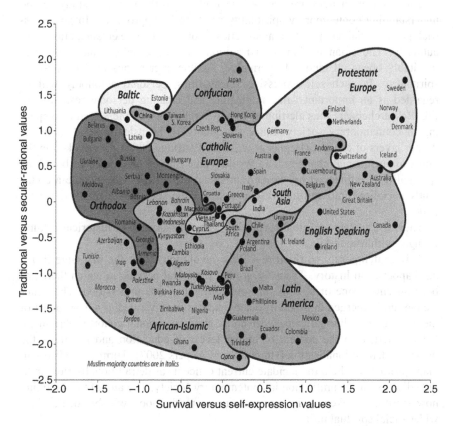

Figure 2.1 Global cultural map: traditional values versus secular-rational values and survival values (2010–2014).

Source: Inglehart and Welzel 2010.

social change as a process of human development, which is producing increasingly humanistic societies that place growing emphasis on human freedom and self- expression'. Postmaterial values focus on one's subjective sense of security, not simply one's objective economic level; and self-expression values are strongly linked with gender equality in political and social life (Inglehart and Welzel 2005).

The 'human development' that these social researchers described in postmaterialistic societies is characterised by a constant focus on agency. Changes that bring larger numbers of people to more fully realise their agentic traits are named human developmental changes (Welzel *et al.* 2003). Researchers suggest that people who place a high emphasis on agency feel that life has more choices and do not feel unduly threatened by suffering (Inglehart and Welzel 2010). Other research has described this state as a 'post-materialist happiness' (Delhey 2010).

These social changes are generating insights into the way that studying and understanding contemporary spirituality needs to be approached. In postindustrial, postmaterial and postsecular societies, people will value emancipation from authority. The emancipation from traditional religious beliefs and authorities inevitably opens all kinds of alternative, flexible expressions of contemporary spirituality. In such self-expressive spiritualities, personal autonomy will be regarded as an important value in shaping and creating personal responses to life. Researchers are thus alerting us to how a relocation of the sacred is happening in contemporary society. Since spirituality is intrinsically residing in the deeper layers of the self (Heelas *et al.* 2005, Partridge 2004), it is evoked in the midst of such social changes. The World Value Survey has indicated both how spirituality is influenced by the current social milieu and why people are currently socialised into spiritual discourse about the self (Hammer 2001; Heelas 2006).

Thus, the current 'spiritual revolution' is a consequence of historical/cultural changes within society.

This contemporary spiritual revival or revolution is not the first time that it has happened in history. There were other historical periods in which there has been an emergence or a 'turn' in how spirituality was understood. This 'subjective turn' emerged in modern society and has been viewed as a by-product of the decline of traditional values, driven by intergenerational cohort replacement. It has emerged in the context of higher levels of education and manifests the theory of detraditionalisation (Houtman and Aupers 2007). Turning to history to map spiritual will help to elucidate current concepts as detraditionalisation, individualisation and pluralisation in contemporary society. The aim of this is to link how spiritual awakening in the transition to motherhood will be located in a wider social spiritual turn.

Second Axial Age

This current spiritual revival has been theorised as a 'Second Axial Age' period of transition. An author with global outreach, such as Karen Armstrong, in her book, *The Great Transformation*, appropriated the term Second Axial Age or (Second Axial Consciousness) – a transition that is similar in character to the First Axial Age. This Second Axial Age traces its roots to the sixteenth and seventeenth centuries. Armstrong asserts that:

> Since the 1970's, there has been a spiritual revival in many parts of the world, and unless there is some kind of spiritual revolution that can keep abreast of our technological genius, it is unlikely that we will save our planet.
>
> (2006, xii)

To understand this current transformation, it is important to return to the First Axial Age period. The Axial Age, or 'Achsenzeit', in German, is a term which was coined by Karl Jaspers in 1949 in his book, *The Origin and Goal of History*. He marked the period from 800 BCE to 200 BCE with an axis at 500 BCE, to indicate the point where 'spiritual foundations of humanity were laid' (Jaspers 1951, 99). He documented how a changed level of consciousness appeared simultaneously at this period in China, India, Persia, Palestine and Greece. Jaspers characterised this period as a time of awakening in humankind to the spiritual impetus in the individual potential of each human being (Jaspers 1963). His philosophy of history had a universal perspective and he was oriented towards discovering the interrelatedness of all unity of meaning within human beings (Jaspers 1951). Thus, the First Axial Age was employed as a construct to establish a sense of connectedness between civilisations. Jaspers proposed the view that there was 'meaning, unity and structure in history' (Jaspers 1951, 98).

Jaspers was influenced by German historicism, but avoided the historicist thinking that tended to discourage active contact between civilisations (Miyang 2009). Some historians have criticised his history of humankind for being 'a chimera', and for not being realistic (Assmann 1988). They considered that without any actual empirical connections between the civilisations of the First Axial Age, what he asserted might only be a coincidence (Köhler 1950).

Consciousness in Jaspers' schema, prior to the First Axial Age, was cosmic, collective, tribal, mythic and ritualistic (Armstrong 2006; Wilber 2007). In the period of the First Axial Age, human beings became conscious of being individual realities. The big psychological/philosophical questions emerged at this period, such as: Who am I? Why are people different? What is being? Why is there anything at all? All these questions were pivotal to the spiritual development occurring, simultaneously, at this period in different parts of the world. The Axial Age began in India, when the ritual reformers started to extract the conflict and aggression from the sacrificial contest. With the concept of *ahimsa*, which means non-injury or non-violence towards all life, Hinduism and Buddhism were born. China's Axial Age developed during the Warring States period, when Confucians, Mohists and Daoists all found ways to counteract widespread lawless and lethal aggression. Thus, Confucianism and Daoism were born. Israel's Axial Age began after the destruction of Jerusalem and the enforced deportation of the exiles to Babylonia, where the priestly writers started to evolve an ideal of reconciliation. Monotheism was conceived in the Middle East. In Greece, where violence was institutionalised by the polis, the essential contribution to the Axial ideal was in the form of tragic theatre. Philosophical rationalism emerged in Ancient Greece (Armstrong 2006). Every single one of these movements began in principle from the unprecedented violence of their time. Every Axial sage at this time (Buddha, Socrates, Confucius, Jeremiah and Ezekiel) encouraged a spirituality of empathy and compassion. Each tradition developed its sacred texts, in which the main golden rule was to abandon egotism, greed, violence and unkindness.

This First Axial Age demanded that people take responsibility for their own actions. Spiritual belief is embedded in the philosophical faith of human beings, which provides the capacity to live with deep questions and the uncertainty of being. *Existenz*, for Jaspers, is a 'choice to be' in the realm of an authentic being. Therefore, *Existenz* is part of a phenomenon of change, of having become different (Jaspers 1967). Jaspers argued that the innate capacity to 'make a choice' of 'conscious living' is the characteristic human capacity which emerged in the First Axial Period.

Jaspers' understandings of the First Axial Age opened the door for scholars to assert that we are today living in the Second Axial Age of spiritual consciousness. Karen Armstrong, for example, traces the roots of this period to the sixteenth and seventeenth centuries of the modern era, when the people of Western Europe began to evolve into a different type of society.

It is difficult to ascertain when a change of axis happens in history and a new Axial Age is born. The origins of the shift marking the beginning of the Second Axial Age may have been as far back as the fourteenth century, with the cultural movement of the Renaissance (Armstrong 2001). The Reformation (sixteenth century), the phenomena of the Enlightenment (1620–1780) and then the Industrial Revolution (1760–1840) were crucial to the economic and social modernisation of Western society. These changes towards a more industrialised world impacted on the spiritual, cultural, economic and social conditions of families. The Age of Reason or Age of Rationalism began with early seventeenth-century philosophy, and it was characterised by a new understanding of the self. The self was conscious, rational, autonomous and universal. The self knew the world through reason and rationality in its objective form. The mode of knowing produced in this period was the objective rational self as 'science'. The only true knowledge was produced and governed by science and reason (Parkinson 1993). The Industrial Revolution manifested the maturity of machine technology and these changes eventually led to a historical period in Western society called modernism (late nineteenth and early twentieth centuries).

The twentieth century was a bloody century with WWI and WWII completely changing the landscape of Europe. At the beginning of the twentieth century, a second scientific revolution changed consciousness forever with Einstein's theory of relativity (1907–1915). Later, by the mid-1920s, the early quantum theory was profoundly reconceived. Revolutionary concepts and discoveries in physics, neurobiology and the scientific study of consciousness started challenging the Newtonian-Cartesian paradigm in Western culture. It is difficult to describe the world by immutable laws, predictable in all its details. Certainly, during the twentieth century this search for certainty has been under siege (e.g. by relativity and quantum mechanics in physics and Godel's theorem in mathematics). In 1979, Douglas R. Hofstadter researched this theorem in his groundbreaking book, *Gödel, Escher, Bach: An Eternal Golden Brain*. One of his conclusions was that the formal system that underlies all mental activity transcends the system that supports it (Hofstadter 1979). These new developments suggested a world where interdependent energy systems are in operation (Bondarenko and Baskin 2014). Carl Jung foresaw these changes, when he wrote:

This is the fateful year for which I have waited more than 25 years. I did not know that it was such a disaster. Although since 1918 I knew that a terrible fire would spread over Europe beginning in the North East, I have no vision beyond 1940 concerning the fate of Europe. This year reminds me of the enormous earthquake in 26 BC that shook down the great temple of Karnak. It was the prelude to the destruction of all temples, because a new time had begun. 1940 is the year when we approach the meridian of the first star in Aquarius. It is the premonitory earthquake of the New Age.[2]

This was a symbolic manifestation of the emotional, psychological and spiritual deconstruction of meaning which was occurring in the middle of the twentieth century. What Carl Jung foresaw were literary, artistic and philosophical changes that would have an impact from the 1960s onwards, into the postmodern period. Deconstructive theories began to manifest in many forms. The 'deconstruction concept' of the postmodern was an abdication from the values of modernity (Norris 1983). French philosopher and sociologist, Jean Francois Lyotard, viewed the 'post-modern condition' as an incredulity towards the 'metanarratives' of modernity: progress and consensus. For Lyotard, consensus is the end of freedom and of thought (Lyotard 1979). Thus, postmodernism became associated with deconstructionist practices that were impacted by the poststructuralism of Jacques Derrida, whose critique of Western logocentrism destabilised and decentred intellectual life (Derrida 1977). The concept of the self that was autonomous in modernity disappeared for a multi-constructed concept of the postmodern self (gender, class, profession, etc.). The interpretation of meaning in a text became multifaceted, with many conflictual perceptions in operation. All these changes have 'shaken and deconstructed' most human spheres. Postmodern thinking allows discrediting, critique and discounting of everything. A 'market' mentality has emerged out of postmodernism, in which things have no longer inherent value, but only exchange value (Rohr 2001). This deconstruction provoked an 'existential anxiety', which stems from stress over freedom and the unknown. This kind of anxiety is a loss of the I-self relationship, related to doubt and the inability to make choices, lack of safety and an expression of sense of meaninglessness. These are feelings of an existential vacuum (emptiness and despair) (Cloninger 2004; 2006; Glass 2003).

The fears and anxiety of the twenty-first century have impacted greatly on maternal ambivalence. Cultural anxiety and expectations have made maternal ambivalence 'the crime that dare not speak its name'.[3] Mothers have real trouble talking about ambivalence and often push these feelings out of consciousness (Almond 2010). Judith Warner's book, *Perfect Madness? Motherhood in the Age of Anxiety* (2006), is a manifesto of postmodern motherhood. The book pictured the image of the mother as a superwoman. In contrast with the 'the feminine mystique' (Friedan 1963) in which women were stay-at-home mothers and fully devoted to motherhood, Warner coined the phrase: 'the mommy mystique', in which mothers must be everything to everyone. The postmodern mother must have and achieve all at any cost. Anxiety and painful emotions are the consequences of the attempts to do motherhood perfectly.

Spirituality has gone through a transition in the modern and postmodern periods. Prior to the postmodern era, Enlightenment thought forced the differentiation and creation of two spheres of reality: religion and rationality. A process of scientific 'colonisation of the life world' (Wilber 2006) was culturally, socially, politically and economically constructed. A technical-scientific rationality grew at the expense of other human spheres of consciousness. Spirituality was often infantilised, ridiculed, denied, repressed and marginalised in modernity. In response, in the postmodern era, a spiritual turn emerged as a pivotal part of the cultural, economic, political and religious change happening in the Western world. A recent study on one of the most worrying issues in contemporary society, climate change, argued that contemporary spirituality cannot be neglected in creating and facilitating a sustainable society (Hedlund-de Witt 2011). In January 2016, United Nations climate chief Christiana Figueres talked to *The Huffington Post* of the inspirational and powerful contribution made by Thich Nhat Hanh to the Paris climate agreement. The Vietnamese Zen Buddhist monk had a deep engagement to bring compassion and insight to the climate crisis with his powerful message, 'Falling in Love with the Earth', submitted to the United Nations in 2014. The emergence of this 'spiritual turn' in contemporary consciousness may be characterised by an emphasis on interconnectedness (Campbell 2007). Thich Nhat Hanh suggests that what it is needed was:

> Love, compassion, generosity, and the insight of our mutual interdependence. We need more than just new technology to protect the planet, we need real community and co-operation. We need to re-establish true communication – true communion – with ourselves, with the Earth, and with one another. What we do as an individual is deeply interconnected with the collective[4]

Figueres believes that he played a pivotal role in helping her to develop the strength, wisdom and compassion needed to forge the unprecedented deal backed by 196 countries.[5] Professor Paul Heelas has researched extensively on spirituality in the postmodern era. In the trilogy of volumes, *The New Age Movement* (Heelas 1996), a co-authored volume, *The Spiritual Revolution* (Heelas *et al.* 2005) and *Spiritualities of Life* (Heelas 2008), he has described the turn as 'a spiritual revolution'. He has argued that the current subjective-life spirituality is 'holistic' in terms of its relationship to nature and self-in-relation rather than a self-in-isolation. This spirituality experiences the need to have 'a profound sense of responsibility for others and the earth' (Heelas 1996, 25). The postmodern self is individualised, but with a difference. This individuality is embedded in the contemporary networked self of the larger whole: family, community, society and environment (Heelas *et al.* 2005). This evolution of consciousness is intrinsically related to the Second Axial transformation that brings a 'global consciousness' to the pattern of contemporary spirituality (Armstrong 2006). It embraces self-actualisation through the service of others (Cook-Greuter 2000). Heelas explored how this 'subjective turn' has impacted on the sociocultural structure of society. Religion has turned into 'subjective-self life spirituality' (Heelas *et al.* 2005).

Religion gives way to spirituality in most subjective spheres of human life: that is, religion is understood subjectively through the lenses of the spiritual self. Heelas sees inner spirituality as having the potential to bring about a world of harmony, peace and bliss (Heelas 1996). An inner change of thinking and feeling can influence how the individual relates more authentically to the world. In general, the contemporary quest for spirituality is often a yearning for a reconstructed interior life (Wade 1999). Heelas has proposed the existence of 'The New Age of Wellbeing', in which the holistic milieu acts as a container for the cultivation and nurturance of subjectivities (Heelas 2008). Subjectivity is the central dynamic of postmodernity (Spiro 1996). In Heelas's findings, two poles of this subjectively appeared:

1   Individuated Subjectivism, in which a self-reliant and self-sufficient individual considers the self as unique and distinct. This subjectivity correlates with possessive individualism and entrepreneurial capitalism.
2   Relational Subjectivism, in which the self operates autonomously but is assisted by others in the tendency to 'go deeper'. Friends, therapists, counsellors are used to talk and assist the journey of the person. It is an interdependent state.

Interestingly, these two different modes of 'subjective turn' can emerge either from external or internal factors (Heelas 2008). This subjective self deeply impacts on the way the spiritual self is understood in postmodernism, since the spiritual self depends profoundly on the historical and cultural background in which it lives. Two counter processes seem to be in operation then in the Second Axial period: individuated and relational subjectivism. Given the global context of the Second Axial period, relational subjectivism will be the 'subjective turn' that is happening in a globalised, inter-netted society. It is in an interdependent state that the individual is exploring their own spirituality. Hence, the significance of mummy blogs for the maternal spiritual journey.

Heelas' latest edited book is a four-volume collection of essays, from around 90 scholars, entitled *Spirituality in the Modern World. Within Religious Tradition and Beyond* (Heelas 2012a). Heelas wrote five of the chapters of this edited book, and his contribution is clearly pointing out at his interests in locating spiritualities of life within cultural developments. Heelas believes in a 'New Age tradition' (Heelas 2012b, 69) in the contemporary world in relation to resources that are neither secular nor sacred. The decline of religious tradition generates spiritual needs that are landing in a 'vacuum' crying out to be filled (Heelas 2012b, 75). Heelas named these spiritual needs in relation to healthcare Contemporary Alternative Medicine (CAM). His research showed that when participants talked about spiritual needs in relation to healthcare, they spoke of CAM and CAM practices such as yoga and meditation. Other participants who were not in any spiritual path, but still engaged in CAM, located their spiritual needs in a 'vacuous', non-explanatory realm unsupported by evidence (Heelas 2012b, 76). This study showed that in general participants reported improvement in a 'subjective well-being' (which was related to the inner experience of the self in this study), when engaged with CAM. This argument on what contributes to healing a person is an important one in the integration of unique spiritual needs that mothers may present in the transition to motherhood in healthcare. Heelas' study highlights a lack of spiritual language in which individuals can articulate such needs, sometimes neither in a sacred nor in a secular way, but in the intersection of the two. Healthcare that provides 'subjective life' bound to holistic themes (involving mind-body-spirit) will be better equipped on the 're/humanization' of the person in the process of healing (Heelas 2012b).

Finding a language of the subjective self in the understanding of contemporary spirituality is crucial. Professor of Religious Studies at the University of Georgia, David Perrin, outlines the concept of the self in the everyday language of the Second Axial Age (Perrin 2007). In his book *Studying Christian Spirituality* (2007, 126), the self is viewed:

1   As the whole human being.
2   As 'something' within us to be discovered.
3   As an identifiable and stable entity but open to change.
4   As a representation but hard to reach and manifest.
5   As a paradox.
6   As culturally defined.

All of these notions of the self are interlinked, and they are used in various disciplines such as philosophy, theology, psychology, sociology or anthropology. The nature of the self is complex. Scholars frequently consider spirituality to be a particular expression of basic human capacities of the self, including language, mind, memory, consciousness and emotions. Thus, it is understood to be intertwined with all the other human capacities. Spiritual capacities contribute, for example, in interpreting and assessing the feelings and images of the psyche (Helminiak 1996). In spiritual terms, the self is treated fundamentally as a manifestation of the human spirit, not independently, but in conjunction with all the psychological, social, cultural, physical and emotional human capacities (Helminiak 1996).

There is a tendency to interpret the spiritual self in a more regressive, pre-rational, romantic perspective (that can fit very well with the understanding of the pre-modern self), and a more progressive way which focuses on inner knowledge and internal growth (Houtman and Aupers 2007). There are dangers in the regression view of the spiritual self. Scholars believe that this 'romantic pre-modern' advocacy of the self abandons and ignores self-responsibility and modern rationality, thus potentially creating a movement towards irrational thinking (Aupers and Houtman 2005; Höllinger 2004; Jacob *et al.* 2009). Such a state of the self can often be regressive, reactionary and deeply narcissistic.

For better or for worse, the Enlightenment has impacted on the contemporary sense of self, and an irreversible shift has been made to the modern self. The Second Axial postmodern self's challenges are those of integration. The postmodern self is always in 'transformation', as it is fragmented. In the latter half of the nineteenth century, a process of breaking up of the personality into fragments began (ego, id, superego, psyche). These were symptoms of the emotional, psychological and spiritual deconstruction of meaning which was occurring. Postmodernism offered the opportunity for the newly discovered spiritual self to explore, reflect, search and be open and flexible. At the same time, the postmodern, Second Axial self must incorporate the 'global consciousness' needed to sustain life on Earth.

Other frameworks, beyond Axial Age theory, account for important influences on the postmodern spiritual self. Processes of detraditionalisation, de-institutionalisation, pluralisation and individualisation are having a profound impact on spirituality. It is essential to consider these movements, so as to understand how they are affecting contemporary spirituality.

Detraditionalisation, individualisation and pluralisation

Postindustrial societies are characterised by an increase in emancipation from traditional external authority. In 1913, the sociologist Georg Simmel foresaw these changes when he wrote:

> The general European consensus is that the era of the Italian Renaissance created what we call individuality. By this is meant a state of inner and external liberation of the individual from the communal forms of the Middle Ages, forms which had constricted the pattern of his life, his activities, and his fundamental impulses through homogenising groups. These had, as it were, allowed the boundaries of the individual to become blurred, suppressing the development of personal freedom, of intrinsic uniqueness, and of the sense of responsibility for one's self.
>
> (1971, 217–218)

In Europe, the process of secularisation and detraditionalisation is a central feature of the changes to which small attitudes shown in the European Value Study.[6] Three important studies have reported this change in the last 30 years, and are under insightful titles: in 1984, *The Silent Turn* (Kerkhofs and Rezsohazy 1984); in 1992, *The Accelerated Turn* (Kerkhofs *et al.* 1992); and in 2000, *Lost Certainty* (Dobbelaere *et al.* 2000).

Professor Lieven Boeve, in his book *Interrupting Tradition*, argues that Europe is not secular, but postsecular, in the sense that among the younger generation (18–29 years old), there is an increase in 'believing without belonging'. This 'detraditionalisation' affects how the traditions are interrupted and not passed on from generations to generations (Boeve 2006). By 'detraditionalisation' he meant the erosion of tradition in religion and society.

Secularisation is the most accurate term to describe a shift in the institutional location of religion and spirituality. As observed by the French sociologist Danielle Hervieu-Leger, this process of 'exiting from religion' is not to be equated with the renunciation of belief. Secularisation of belief is not the end of belief, but the movement by which the elements of belief break free of the structures prescribed by religious institutions (Hervieu-Leger 2001). Today, self-identity is constructed within a plural spiritual market (Boeve 2007).

The dual processes of detraditionalisation and secularisation will lead to 'an individuation of faith', thus yielding religious and spiritual plurality. The outcome of this plurality in the postmodern context is that every narrative or experience has its own legitimacy and validity. In all domains of lifeworld (politics, economy, leisure, education, relationships, art and science) there is no longer a universal 'truth'. There are simply perspectives and many 'realities' (Boeve and Lambert 2001). This turn to personal narrative influences how people develop a new type or types of spiritualities that are based on personal experiences, instead of traditional forms of religion. Sociologist Zygmunt Bauman, in his book *Postmodernity and its Discontents*, explored how this pluralisation is also a 'pluralisation of choices'. In postmodern societies, such pluralisation often provokes an 'anxiety of freedom', in contrast with the 'comforts of certainty' of the modern period (Bauman 1997). As Bauman puts it: 'the hub of postmodern life strategy is not identity building, but the avoidance of being fixed' (1995, 89). In this sense of liberation, individuals are required to negotiate a fragmented, pluralised and ambiguous social order by themselves (Honneth 2004). The ultimate truth does not exist in postmodernity. Therefore, the gods and the institutions that stand for this idea will be discarded for the postmodern individual. The ambivalence of motherhood identity is fuelled by a wider social ambivalence.

In this context, Lieven coined the term 'cultural apophaticism' to describe the soul of this shift of detraditionalisation and pluralisation in contemporary society (Boeve 2006). Cultural apophaticism is an attempt to describe the sacred by negation. Thus the 'grand, classic narratives and stories' – whether religious, social or political – have lost their appeal and credibility (Boeve and Lambert 2001). The loss of these master narratives has provoked three shifts in identity in the postmodern era: the plurality of the postmodern condition, the radical particularity and contextuality of one's own narrative, and the heterogeneity that precipitates a specific contemporary critical consciousness (Boeve 1997).

Irish philosopher, Richard Kearney, reconceived the postmodern condition for the twenty-first century by describing a movement called 'anatheism'. In his book *Anatheism: Returning to God after God*, he described a position between, before and beyond the division of theism and atheism. Kearney's work is an attempt to name the twenty-first century spiritual intersection by expressing 'another word for another way of seeking and sounding the things we consider sacred but can never fully fathom or prove' (2010, 3). This attempt is not a new secularism, atheism or religion. Thus, anatheism is a hermeneutical dialectic between theism and atheism and the non-knowing in between. This non-knowing stance is crucial in the anatheistic paradigm. There is an uncertainty in engaging with the non-knowing, and there is an even greater challenge in trying to name it. Heelas's healthcare research showed the difficulty of expressing spiritual needs in a sacred or in a secular way, which demonstrated the lack of spiritual language in the intersection of the two. Kearney's anatheism cut across all familiar borders: theistic-atheistic, Western-non-Western, sacred-secular, but retained 'a mystical ground of what is most fundamental in each religion and which is not easily translated into language but rather into profound silence' (Kearney 2010, 179). This mystical ground is apophatic in nature similarly with Boeve's 'cultural apophaticism' to describe the spiritual shift in contemporary society (Boeve 2006).

Boeve concludes by reflecting on how this existential turn manages to create a dualist society in which a split occurs. On the one hand is the self-indulgent, obsessed reality of enjoying the goods things in life, and on the other hand is existential insecurity (Boeve 1997). Undoubtedly, this split in society impacts on maternal identity. This postmodern society of 'freedom and choices' poses a real conundrum in motherhood. Contemporary women have fundamentally changed from having maternal destiny to maternal choice. The implications of this shift are both freeing (women are more in the public sphere) and problematic (women's lives and responsibilities in the private sphere are intact). The problem is that those private responsibilities are viewed now as women's 'free' choice. The choices women make are not 'free' choices but are choices within gender constraints (Slaughter 2012).

Bauman captures this predicament of the postmodern individual with the phrase 'having one's cake and eating it' (1997, 182). The individuality of the free is threatened by freedom itself. The most difficult task today is to make the 'right decision' with no consequences: to be able to have freedom without anxiety (Bauman 1997). The acclaimed philosopher and sociologist, Renata Salecl, has explored what she called: 'the tyranny of choice'. She discovered how, paradoxically, in this climate of freedom, there are great feelings of anxiety, guilt and inadequacy and how, like products on a supermarket shelf, our identities seem to be there for the choosing (Salecl 2011). Inevitably in this context, spirituality has often been transformed into a matter of personal choice: personal consumption on personal terms, in response to personal desires grounded in personal authority (Finnegan 2009).

The challenge that society is presented with, in terms of postmodern spirituality, is how the spirituality being discussed engages with the market place in integrity. Carrete and King, in their book, *Selling Spiritualities*, clearly state how different modes of spiritualities are sold as a panacea for the 'mind, body and spirit' revolution. Spirituality has been appropriated for corporate bodies to maintain and extend the market place (Carrete and King 2004). The main challenge is to reclaim and conserve authentic spiritual literacy (Carrete and King 2004).

In view of the historical and cultural landscape of the evolution of spirituality, it is crucial to consider how these changes can be incorporated into the study of contemporary spirituality in the transition to motherhood. The study of spirituality is inevitably embedded in the historical and cultural trends discussed above. As previously mentioned, in light of the forces of detraditionalisation, individualisation and pluralisation of society, spirituality is obliged to study the 'subjective, inner self' in terms of an anthropological study of the 'spiritual self'. Second Axial postmodern spirituality seeks to be in dialogue with all dimensions of the being. Therefore, the study of spirituality needs to be a multidisciplinary and interdisciplinary exploration of the nature of the human subject. Due to the complexity, many disciplines must be engaged in the study of spirituality. Disciplines such as psychology and anthropology can enhance the comprehension of the human spiritual aspects. Spirituality is at the heart of an individual's psychological being. Many studies have researched, and continuing researching, how people are mainly cultural and spiritual beings, and how spirituality is a necessary condition for a psychology of human existence (Fabricatore *et al.* 2000; Koenig 1998; 2009; Pargament 1997; Sue *et al.* 1999).

Notes

1 You can view the surveys online here: www.worldvaluessurvey.org/WVSContents.jsp.
2 Excerpt from a letter written by Carl Jung to his friend, H. G. Baynes on 12 August 1940 (Jung 1973).
3 Paraphrase of Oscar Wilde, who referred to homosexuality as the crime that dare not speak its name in the nineteenth century (Douglas 1892).
4 The full message submitted to the United Nations can be read here: http://newsroom. unfccc.int/1758.aspx.
5 To read the full article, see: www.huffingtonpost.com/entry/thich-nhat-hanh-paris-climate.
6 For more on the European Value Study, see: www.europeanvaluesstudy.eu/.

References

Almond, B. 2010. *The Monster Within. The Hidden Side of Motherhood.* Oakland, USA: University of California Press.
Armstrong, K. 2001. *The Battle for God: Fundamentalism in Judaism, Christianity and Islam.* London: HarperCollins Publishers.
Armstrong, K. 2006. *The Great Transformation: The Beginning of Our Religious Traditions.* New York: Anchor Books.
Assmann, A. 1988. 'Jaspers's Achsenzeit, oder: Schwierigkeiten mit der Zentralperspective in der Geschichte'. In *Karl Jaspers – Denken Zwischen Wissenschaft, Politik und Philosophie*, edited by D. Harth, 187–205. Stuttgart, Germany: Metzler.
Aupers, S., and Houtman, D. 2005. 'Reality Sucks: On Alienation and Cybergnosis'. In *Cyberspace – Cyberethics – Cybertheology*, edited by E. Borgman, S. Van Erp, and H. Haker, 81–90. London: SCM.
Bauman, Z. 1995. *Life in Fragments. Essays in Postmodern Morality.* Oxford, UK: Blackwell Publishers.
Bauman, Z. 1997. *Post Modernity and its Discontents.* Cambridge, UK: Polity Press.
Boeve, L. 1997. 'Critical Consciousness in the Post-Modern Condition'. *Philosophy and Theology* 10(2):449–468.

Boeve, L. 2003. *Interrupting Tradition*. Leuven, Belgium: Peeters Publishers.

Boeve, L. 2006. 'Negative Theology and Theological Hermeneutics: The Particularity of Naming God'. *Journal of Philosophy and Scripture* 3(2):1.

Boeve, L. 2007. 'Europe in Crisis: A Question of Belief or Unbelief? Perspectives from the Vatican'. *Modern Theology* 23(2):205–227.

Boeve, L., and Lambert, L. 2001. *Sacramental Presence in a Postmodern Context*. Leuven, Belgium: Leuven University Press.

Bondarenko, D., and Baskin, K. 2014. *The Axial Ages of World History: Lessons for the 21st Century*. Litchfield Park, USA: Emergent Publications.

Campbell, C. 2007. *The Easternization of the West. A Thematic Account of Cultural Change in the Modern Era*. Boulder, USA: Paradigm Publishers.

Carrete, J., and King, R. 2004. *Selling Spiritualities: The Silent Takeover of Religion*. Oxfordshire, UK: Routledge Publications.

Cloninger, R. 2004. *Feeling Good: The Science of Well Being*. New York: Oxford University.

Cloninger, R. 2006. 'The Science of Well-Being: An Integrated Approach to Mental Health and its Disorders'. *World Psychiatry* 5:71–76.

Cook-Greuter, S. 2000. 'Mature Ego Development: A Gateway to Ego Transcendence?'. *Journal of Adult Development* 7(4):227–240.

Delhey, J. 2010. 'From Materialist to Post-Materialist Happiness? National Affluence and Determinants of Life Satisfaction in Cross-National Perspective'. *Social Indicators Research* 97(1):65–84.

Derrida, J. 1977. *Of Grammatology*. Baltimore, USA: John Hopkins University Press.

Dobbelaere, K., Elchardus, M., Kerkhofs, J., Voyé, L., and Bawin-Legros, B. eds 2000. *Verloren Zekerheid: De Belgen en hun Waarden, Overtuigingen en Houdingen (Lost Certainty)*. Tielt, Belgium: Lannoo.

Douglas, A. 1892. 'Two Loves'. *The Chameleon Magazine*. December.

Fabricatore, A., Handal, P., and Fenzel, L. 2000. 'Personal Spirituality as a Moderator of the Relationship between Stressors and Subjective Well-Being'. *Journal of Psychology & Theology* 28:221–228.

Finnegan, J. 2009. *The Audacity of Spirit*. Dublin: Veritas Publications.

Friedan, B. 1963. *The Feminine Mystique*. New York: Norton.

Gibson, J. 2009. *A Reenchanted World. The Quest for a New Kinship with Nature*. New York: Metropolitan Books.

Glass, G. 2003. *Anxiety – Animal Reactions and Embodiment of Meaning. Nature and Narrative. Introduction to the New Philosophy of Psychiatry*. Oxford, UK: University Press.

Hammer, O. 2001. *Claiming Knowledge: Strategies of Epistemology from Theosophy to the New Age*. Leiden, The Netherlands: Brill.

Hedlund-de Wit, A. 2011. 'The Rising Culture and Worldview of Contemporary Spirituality: A Sociological Study of Potentials and Pitfalls for Sustainable Development'. *Ecological Economics* 70:1057–1065.

Heelas, P. 1996. *The New Age Movement: The Celebration of the Self and the Sacralization of Modernity*. Oxford, UK: Blackwell.

Heelas, P. 2006. 'Challenging Secularization Theory: The Growth of "New Age" Spiritualities of Life'. *Hedgehog Review* 8:46–58.

Heelas, P. 2008. *Spiritualities of Life: New Age Romanticism and Consumptive Capitalism*. Oxford, UK: Wiley-Blackwell.

Heelas, P. 2012a. 'On Making Some Sense of Spirituality'. In *Spirituality in the Modern World. Within Religious Tradition and Beyond,* edited by P. Heelas, 3–37. London: Routledge.

Heelas, P. 2012b. ' "New Age" Spirituality as "Tradition" of Healthcare'. In *Spirituality in Healthcare,* edited by M. Cobb, C. Puchalski, and B. Rumbold, 69–76. Oxford, UK: Oxford University Press.

Heelas, P., Woodhead, L., Seel, B., Szerszynski, B., and Tusting, K. 2005. *The Spiritual Revolution: Why Religion is Giving Way to Spirituality.* Oxford, UK: Wiley-Blackwell.

Helminiak, D. 1996. *The Human Core of Spirituality: Mind as Psyche and Spirit.* New York: State University of New York Press.

Hervieu-Leger, D. 2001. 'The Twofold Limit of the Notion of Secularisation'. In *Peter Berger and the Study of Religion,* edited by L. Woodhead, P. Heelas, and D. Martin, 112–125. London and New York: Routledge.

Hofstadter, D. 1979. *Gödel, Escher, Bach: An Eternal Golden Brain.* New York: Harvester Press.

Höllinger, D. 2004. 'Damned for God's Glory: William James and the Scientific Vindication of Protestant Culture'. In *Re-experiencing Varieties: William James and a Science of Religion,* edited by W. Proudfoot, 9–30. New York: Columbia University Press.

Honneth, A. 2004. 'Organized Self-Realization. Some Paradoxes of Individualization'. *European Journal of Social Theory* 7(4):463–478.

Houtman, D., and Aupers, S. 2007. 'The Spiritual Turn and the Decline of Tradition: The Spread of Post-Christian Spirituality in Fourteen Western Countries (1981–2000)'. *Journal for the Scientific Study of Religion* 46(3):305–320.

Inglehart, R., and Welzel, C. 2005. *Modernization, Cultural Change, and Democracy. The Human Development Sequence.* New York: Cambridge University Press.

Inglehart, R., and Welzel, C. 2008. 'The Role of Ordinary People in Democratization'. *Journal of Democracy* 19(1):26–140.

Inglehart, R., and Welzel, C. 2010. 'Changing Mass Priorities: The Link between Modernization and Democracy'. *Perspectives on Politics* 8:551–567.

Jacob, J., Jovic, E., and Brinkerhoff, M. 2009. 'Personal and Planetary Well-Being: Mindfulness Meditation, Pro-environmental Behavior and Personal Quality of Life in a Survey from the Social Justice and Ecological Sustainability Movement'. *Social Indicators Research* 93:275–294.

Jaspers, K. 1949/2011. *The Origin and Goal of History.* New York: Routledge Revivals.

Jaspers, K. 1951. *Way to Wisdom. An Introduction to Philosophy.* New Haven, USA: Yale University Press.

Jaspers, K. 1963. *Philosophy and the World. Selected Essays and Lectures.* Chicago, USA: University of Chicago.

Jaspers, K. 1967. *Philosophical Faith and Revelation.* Glasgow, UK: Harper & Row.

Jung, C. 1973. *Letters of C. G. Jung: Volume I, 1906-1950.* New Jersey, USA: Princeton University Press.

Kearney, R. 2010. *Anatheism: Returning to God after God.* New York: Columbia University Press.

Kerkhofs, J., Dobbelaere, K., and Voyé, L. eds 1992. *De Versnelde Ommekeer: De Waarden van Vlamingen, Walen en Brusselaars in de Jaren Negentig. (The Accelerated Turn).* Tielt, Belgium: Lannoo.

Kerkhofs, J., and Rezsohazy, R. eds 1984. *De Stille Ommekeer: Oude en Nieuwe Waarden in het België van de Jaren Tachtig (The Silent Turn).* Tielt, Belgium: Lannoo.

Koenig, H. 1998. *Handbook of Religion and Mental Health.* New York: Academic Press.

Koenig, H. 2009. 'Research on Religion, Spirituality, and Mental Health: A Review'. *Canadian Journal of Psychiatry* 54(5):283–291.

Köhler, O. 1950. 'Das Bild der Menschheitsgeschichte bei Karl Jaspers'. *Saeculum* 1:477–486.

Lyotard, J. 1979. *La Condition Postmoderne: Rapport sur la Savoir (The Postmodern Condition: A Report on Knowledge).* Paris: Minuit.

Miyang, C. 2009. 'The Global History of Humankind in Karl Jaspers' Existenz'. *An International Journal for Philosophy, Religion, Politics, and the Arts* 4:20–25.

Norris, C. 1983. *The Deconstructive Turn.* London: Methuen.

Pargament, K. 1997. *Psychology of Religion and Coping: Theory, Research, Practice.* New York: Guilford Press.

Parkinson, G. ed. 1993. *The Renaissance and the 17th Century Rationalism.* London and New York: Routledge.

Partridge, C. 2004. *The Re-enchantment of the West (Vol. 1): Understanding Popular Occulture.* London: Continuum.

Perrin, D. 2007. *Studying Christian Spirituality.* Oxford, UK: Routledge.

Rohr, R. 2001. *Hope Against Darkness: The Transforming Vision of Saint Francis of Assisi in an Age of Anxiety.* Denver, USA: St Anthony Messenger Press.

Salecl, R. 2011. *The Tyranny of Choice.* Croydon, UK: Profile Books.

Simmel, G. 1971. 'Freedom and the Individual'. In *George Simmel on Individuality and Social Forms*, edited by D. N. Levine, 217–226. London: The University of Chicago Press.

Slaughter, A. 2012. 'Why Women Still Can't Have it All'. *The Atlantic Monthly.* www.theatlantic.com/magazine/archive/2012/07/why-women-still-cant-have-it-all/309020/.

Spiro, M. 1996. 'Postmodernist Anthropology, Subjectivity, and Science: A Modernist Critique'. *Comparative Studies in Society and History* 38(4):759–780.

Sue, D., Bingham, R., Porche-Burke, L., and Vasquez, M. 1999. 'The Diversification of Psychology: A Multicultural Revolution'. *American Psychologist* 54:1061–1069.

Tarnas, R. 2007. *Cosmos and Psyche. Intimations of a New World View.* New York: Plume.

Wade, C. 1999. *Spiritual Marketplace: Baby Boomers and the Remaking of American Religion.* Princeton, USA: Princeton University Press.

Warner, J. 2006. *Perfect Madness? Motherhood in the Age of Anxiety.* New York: Riverhead Books.

Welzel, C., Ronald, I., and Hans-Dieter, K. 2003. 'The Theory of Human Development: A Cross-Cultural Analysis'. *European Journal of Political Research* 42(2):341–380.

Wilber, K. 2006. *Integral Spirituality: A Startling New Role for Religion in the Modern and Post-Modern World.* Boston, USA: Shambhala.

Wilber, K. 2007. *The Integral Vision: A Very Short Introduction to the Revolutionary Integral Approach to Life, God, the Universe, and Everything.* Boston, USA: Shambhala and York: Metropolitan Books.

3 Spirituality and interdisciplinary partners

Spirituality and psychology

The historical and social intersection between spirituality and psychology is crucial in the understanding of the psycho-spiritual paradigm.

During the twentieth century, an acceptance of transpersonal theories and spiritual experience has been incorporated into clinical practice. In 1912, Carl Jung expanded Freud's psychoanalytic understanding of the structure of the psyche to include a spiritual wholeness framework. Jung was the first clinician who attempted to legitimise a spiritual approach in the development of the psyche (Jung 1967). Abraham Maslow followed with spirituality studies of persons whom he considered to be 'self-actualised' (Maslow 1962). Lukoff (1985), Grof and Grof (1989) and Agosin (1992) have all made their contribution to analysing transpersonal experiences, using language such as 'spiritual emergence' and 'spiritual emergency' (Grof and Grof 1989). They have researched out-of-body experiences, near-death experiences, ultimate values, spiritual development and deep healing.

Transpersonal psychology study of spirituality

Transpersonal psychology is a key subfield of psychology which has advanced the study of spirituality. This approach to psychology is interested in the experiences of the individual's sense of identity and explores beyond the autonomous self to psyche, life, the cosmos and humankind (Gollnick 2005). Therefore, transpersonal theory proposes that there are developmental stages beyond the adult ego, which involve phenomena outside the boundaries of the ego (Kasprow and Bruce 1999).

The notion of 'transpersonal' was introduced by the Harvard philosopher and psychologist, William James, at the beginning of the twentieth century (Vich 1988). He took the spiritual dimension seriously in the development of human beings. William James's classic text, *The Varieties of Religious Experience* (1902/1985, 42) claimed: 'Religious genius (experience) should be the primary topic in the study of religion, rather than religious institutions – since institutions are merely the social descendant of genius'. The investigation of mystical experience was a constant interest throughout his academic career. James's view was that spiritual experiences would be mediated by their effect on people, rather than being transmitted by a particular theoretical, cultural or religious orientation. He believed that spirituality was to 'come face to face with facts which no instinct or reason can ever know' (James 1902/1885, 307). Those who have had spiritual experiences are 'illuminated' and are usually profoundly changed in their views. He called this universal type of experience 'a connection with the divine' (James 1902/1985, 42). He felt that these experiences were rooted in mystical states of consciousness that revealed transcendence of normal reality:

> It makes a tremendous emotional and practical difference to one whether one accepts the universe in the drab discoloured way of stoic resignation to necessity, or with the passionate happiness of Christian saints. The difference is as great as that between passivity and activity, as that between the defensive and the aggressive mood. Gradual as are the steps by which an individual may grow from one state into the other, many as are the intermediate stages which different individuals represent, yet when you place the typical extremes beside each other for comparison, you feel that two discontinuous psychological universes confront you, and that in passing from one to the other a 'critical point' has been overcome.
>
> (James 1909/1977, 41)

In his classic text, he clearly expressed the process of reaching changed states of consciousness. His mystical attributes – ineffability, noetic quality, transience and passivity – are encapsulated in the above extract from his book. The spiritual, transcendental experience is ineffable in the sense of how difficult it is to relate it with words and language, because it is caught between two shades of meaning. The noetic quality of the experience refers to the Greek word *gnosis*, meaning knowledge. This aspect indicates how mystical insight will generate a new perception of the universe or cosmos. The transient character of this state indicates how short and intense such experiences are and how difficult it is to grasp them. Passivity is used by James to describe the ways in which the mystical experience occurs: in its greatest intensity, it occurs without the active will of the individual. In transpersonal experience, loss of clear ego-boundaries is part of the experience.

Others, such as the transcendentalist Emerson, described such experiences thus: 'Standing on the bare ground, – my head bathed by the blithe air, and uplifted into infinite space, – all mean egotism vanishes' (Emerson 2011, 4), while the mystic, Teresa of Avila, called these glimpses of ultimate mystery, 'a state of great quiet and deep satisfaction' (Teresa of Avila 2002, 306).

While William James pioneered the capturing of descriptions of the spiritual experience, through time, stages were standardised to describe spiritual experience. Scholars such as Evelyn Underhill mapped out her own stages of the mystic's journey into five phases: awakening of self, purgation of self, illumination, the dark night of the soul and the unitative life (Underhill 2011).

Currently, the term 'mysticism' is open to a wide academic debate, as it has only been around since 1736. Many scholars are critical of William James' mystical schema. It is difficult to conceptualise these stages, as they are non-rational. James's stages may seem too reductionist and rational in nature (Otto 1931). Other scholars believe that Jamesian ideas did not acknowledge the cultural context of the person having the experiences, and such experiences cannot be disassociated from so-called normal conscious states (Stace 1960; Zaehner 1957). The study of mysticism aims at understanding the practices, discourses and experiences associated with human transformation. William James made the pioneering attempt to understand human experience through his own phenomenology of mystical experiences.

The transpersonal concept is concerned with the awareness or consciousness states that are no longer confined exclusively to the individual ego. Current academic dialogue has described these states as related to self-identity, being and consciousness in which self-identity becomes integrated into a 'deeper' or 'higher' perspective of the world (Vaughan 2005).

The questions that arise in the transpersonal context are: is motherhood a loss of boundary of the individual ego? Is the transition to motherhood a 'natural' experience that force mothers to go beyond the individual ego? Can mothers conceptualise or even name any transpersonal experiences? What happens beyond the ego experiences once you enter into it? Many times, growing or transcending beyond the ego can provoke pathological reactions as defensive responses. Therefore, it is important to analyse the transpersonal phenomenon in the study of spirituality in relation to the transition to motherhood.

Transpersonal psychology in essence, as explained above, is interested in forces which are greater than the egoic self.[1] The transpersonal approach values spirituality and places it at the core of its theories. Since the investigation of mystical experience was constant throughout the career of William James, arguably he is the father of transpersonal psychology.

At the same time, it is important to note that transpersonal psychology is also a study of consciousness within the individual. These experiences (the experiences of the mothers interviewed) relate to growing in consciousness in which the perception of self is expanded beyond the ego (Caplan *et al.* 2003).

Humanistic psychology study of spirituality

Humanistic psychology, which arose in the mid-twentieth century, is a second central subfield of psychology for investigating spirituality. The humanistic approach investigates human beings in terms of the meaning, values, freedom and potential, all of which are central to the spirituality of the individual. Humanistic theorists have understood spirituality as a fundamental capacity in human beings: a capacity that is embedded in the spiritual nature of the human person. The concentration camp survivor and academic, Victor Frankl, saw the human capacity for conscience as a sort of 'unconscious spirituality' (Frankl 2006), different from the instinctual unconscious. He argued that spirituality was an innate capacity for creating a framework of the ultimate meaning of one's life. By contrast, the humanist psychologist Carl Rogers viewed human beings as energy fields 'different from the sum of their parts' (1980, 4), actualising potentials in the process of becoming. Rogerian theory referred to spirituality as both the existence and the experience of integrality, which manifests itself as increased awareness of the interconnectedness of people and environment (Rogers 1980).

In an equivalent manner, the educational psychologist Maslow described movement towards self-actualisation as making the 'growth choice instead of the fear choice' many times and argued that spirituality provides a vision of what one can grow towards (Maslow 1964, 159). When he wrote the essay that launched the *Journal of Transpersonal Psychology*, he was a humanistic who had glimpsed a vision of humankind that reunited the spiritual and mystical traditions. Maslow announced a revolution, a shift in the modernist foundations of society and science at the time. His 'new image of humankind' was not confined by modernism or eroded by postmodernism. Before the Grofs (1976) identified transpersonal experiences, Maslow wrote extensively about peak experiences (Maslow 1962).

He believed that these peak experiences can generate deep changes at many levels of the human self-concept. In this regard, Maslow discussed early in the development of peak experiences how these experiences can change identity dramatically. For Maslow, identity was the most fundamental standard for what concerns human beings, because everyone evaluates almost everything against their 'self-concept'. Going through these peak experiences can provoke a profound shift in consciousness in the individual (Friedman and Hartelius 2013, 586).

Building on Maslow's self-actualisation concept, Hungarian psychologist Mihaly Csikszentmihalyi described the concept of 'flow'. Self-actualised people experience this 'flow' as state of mind when they are using their full potential, completely immersed in an activity without being conscious of time, or anything else. Self-actualised people often experience flow, as well as peak experiences. Csikszentmihalyi distinguished peak experiences as external occurrences and 'flow' as an internal mental process (Csikszentmihalyi 1994). Flow as an internal mental process can challenge anxiety, distress and uneasiness in human identity.

Similarly, the American existential psychologist Rollo May believed in the realisation of the self through the confrontation of anxiety-creating experiences. He held that it is in anxiety experienced as a young child that the self comes into being with an 'existential anxiety' (Rollo 2015). He viewed creativity as the authentic, existential and self-actualising, transcending state that, as spirituality, will transcend human egocentrism (Rollo 1994).

Robert Assagioli's psychosynthesis mode is perhaps the clearest map of spiritual growth within a humanistic framework. Assagioli insisted that there are 'higher urges within man which tend to make him grow towards greater realisations of his spiritual essence' (Rollo 1994, 193). Assagioli created a notion of psychology broad enough to deal with spiritual development. He explains: 'We are not attempting to force upon psychology a philosophical, theological or metaphysical position, but essentially we include within the study of psychological facts all those which may be related to the higher urges' (Rollo 1994, 194). Professor David Perrin has aimed at creating a humanistic understanding of spirituality, as has been identified by the above theorists, that is common to all humans, independent of culture, religion or belief. In his book, *Studying Christian Spirituality*, he defined spirituality as: 'a lived experience of conscious involvement in the project of life integration through self-transcendence toward the ultimate value one perceives' (2007, 20).

Perrin outlined four elements that enhance the understanding of spirituality from a humanistic approach and create the necessity to study it seriously in the academia. The first element is that spirituality is a human spiritual nature. The search for meaning, values, reflection and purpose in life, are some of the spiritual innate qualities that humans possess. The second element is the capacity for transcendence and self-transcendence. These capacities are interlinked with intimacy, relationships with others and ultimately, with the planet. It is also about the awareness that reality is beyond what can be seen or touched. The third element is that spirituality is a 'lived reality', in which attitudes, practices, rituals and behaviours describe the daily lives of people. Chapter 6 of this book explores in depth this lived spiritual reality. The fourth and final element is the academic study of spirituality.

Motherhood involves how people live out their reality: with family life, the workplace, public life, health or ethics. Perrin believed that all those aspects of life need to be studied seriously in academia. He also encouraged inquiry into the dynamics of the spiritual life, engaging other disciplines such as psychology, anthropology or sociology (Perrin 2007).

In the humanistic understanding of spirituality, the 'spirit' transcends the 'ego' and the 'psyche'. According to Perrin, the 'spirit' of spirituality may have nothing to do with God, the Holy Spirit or the Divine Spirit. He felt that while these concepts are significant in Christian, Islamic, Jewish and even indigenous spirituality, they do not encompass the whole understanding of innate humanistic understanding of the concept of 'spirit' (Perrin 2007).

Perrin (2007) believes that human spirit is in human consciousness as a fundamental dimension of human beings. In these terms, spirituality is understood as an innate, human capacity aligned with physical and emotional capacities. Some critiques on Perrin's understanding of spirituality are related to the physical or emotional capacities that he believed to be innate in the development of spirituality. It is important to note that research has been done with individuals who have altered either their physical or emotional or both capacities. There may be an understanding that the concepts or capacities to achieve a development of spirituality are too sophisticated and complicated and require a level of awareness which the profoundly mentally or physically handicapped do not have. Professor John Swinton has long researched the spirituality of disability and has developed compassionate and careful pastoral responses to dementia and forgetfulness (Swinton 2012). In his research, he has also examined the spiritual experiences of people with enduring mental health issues and the reasons why psychiatrists have tended to neglect or pathologise the spiritual in these particular groups (Swinton 2001).

Swinton has uncovered the significance of spirituality for people with learning disabilities and the importance for this group of people to find a mode of language and a form of self-expression (Swinton 2001). Swinton's research includes the development of a model that through agencies that can train carers and support workers to recognise and meet the spiritual needs of this group of individuals (Swinton 2006; 2007; 2011).

Perrin also describes the three specific characteristics of the 'spirit' in humanistic spirituality. The first characteristic is that the spirit is not an objective phenomenon. He explains how the work of the human spirit can be observable only through the mediation of human action and production. Thus, he believes that it is important to look beyond consciousness into the broadest range of human life with self-reflection (Perrin 2007). The second characteristic is that the spirit can be conscious but also unconscious. The work of the human spirit was to become more conscious of intentions, desires and motivations. Different spiritual capacities will help in this task, such as self-reflection and awareness. Accordingly, the human spirit will grow and mature by getting to know this unconscious part of our spirit and transforming how it affects our lives.

The third and final characteristic is that the spirit involves the deepest dimension of human life. This is related to how human beings need to risk and explore different domains beyond the self. Indeed, new skills are needed to be aware of and embrace the mystery of our own spirit (Perrin 2007).

In the humanistic understanding of spirituality, spirit can be described as the deepest core of humanity. Perrin stated that, 'the spiritual centre is the deepest centre of the person, where the authenticity and love of humans are open to the transcendent' (2007, 22).

Both the transpersonal and humanistic understandings of spirituality are useful for the study of the maternal transition. Within psychology, the transpersonal and humanistic approaches are the only ones that tend to understand and analyse the spiritual dimension of the individual. These approaches understand spirituality as holistic in nature. They look at the whole person and encourage a self-awareness and mindfulness that helps the individual change and grow. They also understand spirituality universally. Anthropologically, human beings may be described as sharing spiritual qualities within themselves independently of where they come from and what religion they profess.

Professor of Humanistic and Transpersonal Psychology, Daniel Helminiak believed that consciousness may be both reflecting and non-reflecting: reflecting because it is intentional, and non-reflecting because it is not directed towards any object. Rather, consciousness is an awareness of subjectivity (Helminiak 1996). Rooted in these ideas of the human consciousness, Helminiak (1996, 57) described the human spirit as, 'that experienced reality that constitutes subjectivity. Spirit is what makes you an aware subject. Spirit is experienced as non-reflecting consciousness'.

Helminiak outlines spiritual development in four principles: the first principle is the authentic self-transcendence that will be facilitated by the second principle of openness. The third principle involves wholeness and integration. This principle involves the whole person and it is often associated with the holistic view that spirituality is adopting in the present time. The last principle is the reflective self-analysis that individuals need to develop in order to achieve a mature spiritual development (Helminiak 1987).

For Helminiak, then, spirituality is fundamentally a matter of human spirit rather than of religious systems and their relationships with supreme beings (Helminiak 1996). He argues that since spirituality deals with the human spirit, the discipline of spirituality must be integrated into the human sciences:

> The peculiar quality of human spirit is its non-reflecting awareness of itself. Because the human spirit is aware of itself and always more than what it has objectified, it is a dynamic reality, characterised by marvel, wonder or question, open ultimately to everything there is to be known and loved.
>
> (Helminiak 1996, 127)

Helminiak acknowledges how human beings are organism, psyche and spirit. He stresses how it is the spirit that subsumes the psyche and the organism, and how the spirit is at the core of what being human means. The human organism and the human psyche are human precisely because they are under the influence of the human spirit. Thus, he coined the axiom: 'the human psyche is enspirited' (Helminiak 1996, 141). For Helminiak, it is crucial to appreciate the interaction between the human mind, the psyche and the spirit.

According to Helminiak, the images and messages of the psyche indicate the state of the organism. Deciphering the symbolic expressions of the psyche through phenomena such as dreams is sometimes difficult. Humans do have the capacity to self-transform their patterns of response and reform their personalities. Helminiak believes that embracing such change is the demand of the innate urge for authenticity within the human spirit. Thus, psyche and spirit collaborate in the process of spiritual growth. The collaboration of psyche, organism and spirit is critical to authentic spirituality. Therefore, the explanation of this lived experience or lived spirituality is of deep concern for the understanding and study of spirituality (Helminiak 1996).

Conclusions

The field of psychology studies human behaviour and experience and assists people to clarify their progression and decline across the lifespan. Similarly, spirituality can help people make sense of their own lives. Thus, humanistic/ transpersonal approaches to the study of spirituality value human experience and are equipped to deal with the current cultural/historical changing paradigms of individual identity. These psychological approaches to spirituality provide frameworks to explain the mothers' dynamics of spiritual unfolding in relation to all other aspects of their lives. The turn to transpersonal and humanistic psychology is adaptable to incorporating diverse maternal experiences.

In the next chapter, in order to test the 'Psycho-spiritual paradigm in the transition to motherhood' and to better understand the interaction between spirituality and motherhood, a pilot study was carried out using anthropological, transpersonal and humanistic approaches to spirituality. The next chapter examines the pilot study conducted by interviewing four first-time mothers. The aim of doing this pilot study was to examine what spiritual capacities may emerge in the transition to motherhood and also to test how these interdisciplinary partners help in the study of spirituality in the phenomenon of motherhood.

Note

1 The 'egoic self' is the state of being identified with the ego. It is the power that defends and glorifies the separated self, works for separation, unhealthy autonomy and independence. In psychological terms, the ego is the part of the psyche that experiences the outside world and reacts to it, coming between the primitive drives of the id and the demands of the social environment, represented by the superego.

References

Agosin, T. 1992. 'Psychosis, Dreams and Mysticism in the Clinical Domain'. In *The Fires of Desire,* edited by F. Halligan and J. Shea, 41–65. New York: Crossroad.

Caplan, M., Hartelius G., and Rardin M. 2003. 'Contemporary Viewpoints on Transpersonal Psychology'. *Journal of Transpersonal Psychology* 35(2):143–162.

Csikszentmihalyi, M. 1994. *The Evolving Self: A Psychology for the Third Millennium.* New York: Harper Perennial Press.

Emerson, R. W. 2011. *Nature.* Seattle, USA: Amazon Digital Services, Inc. Kindle Edition.

Frankl, V. 2006. *Man's Searching for Meaning.* Boston, USA: Beacon Press.

Friedman, H., and Hartelius, G. 2013. *The Wiley-Blackwell Handbook of Transpersonal Psychology.* West Sussex, UK: John Wiley & Son Publishers.

Gollnick, J. 2005. *Religion and Spirituality in the Life Cycle.* New Jersey, USA: Peter Lang Publishing.

Grof, S., and Grof, C. 1976. *The Transpersonal Vision: The Healing Potential of Non-Ordinary States of Consciousness.* New York: E. P. Dutton.

Grof, S., and Grof, C. 1989. *Spiritual Emergency: When Personal Transformation Becomes a Crisis.* New York: TarcherPerigee.

Helminiak, D. 1987. *Spiritual Development: An Interdisciplinary Study.* Chicago, USA: Loyola Press.

Helminiak, D. 1996. *The Human Core of Spirituality: Mind as Psyche and Spirit.* New York: State University of New York Press.

James, W. 1902/1985. *The Varieties of Religious Experience.* Cambridge, USA: Harvard University Press.

James, W. 1909/1977. *A Pluralistic Universe.* Cambridge, USA: Harvard University Press.

Jung, C. 1967. 'Symbols of Transformation (1912)'. In *Collected Works, Volume 5,* translated by R. F. C. Hull. Princeton, USA: Princeton University Press.

Kasprow, M., and Bruce, W. 1999. 'A Review of Transpersonal Theory and its Application to the Practice of Psychotherapy'. *Journal of Psychotherapy Practice and
Research* 8(1):12–23.

Lukoff, D. 1985. 'The Diagnosis of Mystical Experiences with Psychotic Features'.
Journal of Transpersonal Psychology 17:155–181.

Maslow, A. 1962. *Toward a Psychology of Being.* Princeton, USA: Van Nostrand.

Maslow, A. 1964. *Religions, Values, and Peak Experiences.* Columbus: Ohio State
University Press.

Otto, R. 1931. *The Idea of the Holy: An Inquiry into the Non-Rational Factor in the Idea
of the Divine and its Relation to the Rational.* London: Oxford University Press.

Perrin, D. 2007. *Studying Christian Spirituality.* Oxford, UK: Routledge Publishing.

Rogers, C. 1980. *A Way of Being.* Boston, USA: Houghton Mifflin.

Rollo, M. 1994. *The Courage to Create.* New York: W.W. Norton and Company.

Rollo, M. 2015. *The Meaning of Anxiety.* New York: W.W. Norton and Company.

Stace, W. 1960. *Mysticism and Philosophy.* Philadelphia, USA: J.B. Lippincott.

Swinton, J. 2001. *Spirituality in Mental Health Care: Rediscovering a Forgotten Dimension.* London: Jessica Kingsley Publishers.

Swinton, J. 2006. 'Identity and Resistance: Why Spiritual Care Needs "Enemies"'.
Journal of Clinical Nursing 15(7):918–928.

Swinton, J. 2007. '"Forgetting Whose We are": Theological Reflections on Successful
Aging, Personhood and Dementia'. *Journal of Religion, Disability and Health*
11(1):37–63.

Swinton, J. 2011. '"Whose Story Am I?" Theology, Spirituality and Profound Intellectual
Disabilities'. *Journal of Religion Disability and Health* 15(1):5–19.

Swinton, J. 2012. *Dementia: Living in the Memories of God.* Grand Rapids, USA: Eerd-
mans.

Teresa of Avila. 2002. *The Complete Works of St. Teresa of Jesus.* London, New York,
and Harrisburg, USA: Continuum International Publishing Group.

Underhill, E. 2011. *Mysticism: A Study in Nature and Development of Spiritual Consciousness.* Seattle, USA: Amazon Digital Services LLC.

Vaughan. 2005. *Shadows of the Sacred: Seeing through Spiritual Illusions.* Bloomington,
USA: iUniverse.com.

Vich, M. 1988. 'Some Historical Sources for the Term "Transpersonal"'. *Journal of
Transpersonal Psychology* 20:107–110.

Zaehner, R. 1957. *Mysticism: Sacred and Profane: An Inquiry into Some Varieties of
Praeternatural Experiences.* Oxford, UK: Oxford University Press.

4 Testing the psycho-spiritual approach in the transition to motherhood

A pilot study

In this pilot qualitative study, four first-time mothers were interviewed regarding their experiences of birth, the transition to motherhood and the postnatal period. At the time of the interview, all mothers were married, and they were in their 30s. They all had small children; the mean age was three years old. When they were approached, a year had passed since the birth of their babies. Thus, these women had had an 'engagement' with motherhood. In the maternal literature, 'engagement' has been identified as central to the first year of motherhood (Barlow 1997). This first year will lead to a 'transformation' in the social, cultural, physical and emotional context of the women. Since spiritual wellbeing is understood in this study to be intertwined with the physical, social and emotional needs of the mother, the aim of this pilot study was to explore the spiritual transformation experiences that occurred in the liminal space created by the transition to motherhood.

Liminality, spirituality and motherhood

In this pilot study, liminality is understood from an anthropological viewpoint. Liminality comes from the Latin, meaning 'a threshold'. Motherhood is of one of the major life transitions experienced by women: the threshold between womanhood and motherhood. Pregnancy, birth and the transition to motherhood have been found to create conditions that are ritualistic in nature (Lahood 2007). Anthropologically, being on the 'threshold' is existing within two existential planes: a rite of passage. Anthropologist Van Gennep observed three basic stages within rites of passage: the 'preliminal rites' that served to separate the participant from his or her previous world, the liminal or threshold rites, and the postliminal ceremonies of incorporation into a new world (Van Gennep 2004). In motherhood, the prenatal stage can be considered the 'preliminal', as it assists the woman into the threshold and the postpartum as the postliminal rite. Women in this study reported mostly on experiences which correspond to the second stage of the rite of passage: the liminal space. In this space, there are frequent feelings of loss, challenges and disruptions to the existing structure (Turner 1995). It is difficult to determine the length of time of the maternal liminal space as it is unique for every mother.

Key themes

Theme 1: crisis and descent into the underworld

> There is a natural time after child bearing when a woman is considered to be
> of the underworld. She is dusted with its dust, watered by its water, having
> seen into the mystery of life, death, pain and joy during her labour. So, for a
> time *she is 'not here' but rather still 'there'* (researcher's emphasis).
>
> (Estes-Pinkola 1996, 441)

Crisis is a term that can be defined with many different connotations. Its meaning
is a turning point, a condition of instability, and a danger of a dramatic emotional
or circumstantial upheaval in a person's life. In literature, it is the point of the
story at which hostile elements are most tensely opposed to each other. In medicine, it is the point in the course of a serious disease at which a decisive change
occurs, leading either to recovery or to death.[1]

Mythically and archetypally, the descent into the underworld is characterised
by a psychospiritual initiation. In this study, liminality, the underworld and the
unconscious are interchangeable terms that have been used to denote an individual space in which the person undergoes an identity crisis by being faced with
a deep challenge, undergoing a growth experience, entering a transpersonal/
sacred space, undergoes an identity crisis and, has a sense of being an outsider
(Carroll 2003).

In this liminal phase 'in-between' the unconscious and the conscious stages,
the woman is struggling with ambiguity, opposing feelings and paradoxes. The
initiation or emergence has been described by anthropologists as a 'breakthrough' that is often painful, acute, dramatic and one that happens on all levels:
material, spiritual and bodily (Steindl Rast 1985). Once the darkness of the symbolic and archetypal unconscious has been entered, a deconstruction of identity
occurs. In some maternal studies, this experience is identified as a personal crisis
and a type of identity disintegration which can threaten the woman's sense of
self (Darvill *et al.* 2010).

All participants described crisis feelings associated with 'entering the
unknown' and an intense conflict in identity:

> I just had no idea what was going on, what was coming you know, it sounds
> great but you just don't know what you are getting yourself into and then
> here: that's a baby.
>
> (Interviewee 4)

> Yeah sometimes it was teary eyed how hard this is. How am I going to do
> this? How long is this going to last? Where is my life gone? I actually found
> that very difficult. My own needs not be[ing] met. Where am I in this? What
> is happening?
>
> (Interviewee 1)

Parratt and Fahy observed that

> Maternal identity is suspended between the opposites of subjectivity and objectivity and is unable to wholly inhabit either of the two. In the paradoxical nature of liminality, death coexists with birth. In a study into birth, women described their experiences of becoming a mother in terms of 'facing death' and of 'survival'.
>
> (2003)

In this paradoxical place, the transcendent function of the self helps to bridge or remove the gap between subject and object (Miller 2004). There is a symbolic dialogue with the unconscious that the new mother needs to dare to engage with. This dialogue is a form of spiritual emergence, an awakening and a step to a more expansive way of being, in which there is a development of a more profound consciousness (Wilber 1986). In this stage, the awareness of the woman's value system is tested by the vulnerability of her newborn baby. In the fog of this process, she seeks to comprehend what is meaningful in order to achieve adjustments.

A spiritual crisis has been defined as a drastic change in the individual's meaning system (Grof and Grof 1989). A maternal study concluded that the transformation, growth and transition into motherhood are usually mediated by reflective self-acceptance, spiritual perception and increased self-awareness (Akerjordet 2010). Openness to change and to letting go of the old self is one of the foundational factors in integrating a spiritual experience (Bragdon 1993; 2013). Mothers often struggle with change versus rigidity. Feelings of control and perfectionism in the face of the new realities of motherhood were repeatedly related at length in the interviews. Mothers experienced their crisis of no longer having control over anything in life. They tended to rigidify their experiences:

> I don't know. I suppose I had a bit of fear of losing control or not being able to cope or do something. I just started to feel really like I wasn't coping.
>
> It wasn't that I was trying to be a perfect mother or anything. I don't know what it was. I was just too determined to do things the way I thought I wanted to do it.
>
> (Interviewee 1)

Psychologically, control is one of the mechanisms that the ego uses to counteract persecutory anxiety (Searles 1965). Maternal anxiety was also a common and recurrent theme within the narratives of the new mothers in this study. They discussed how they had tried to understand this anxiety and the feelings that it provoked:

> There is the anxiety in there as well. I am trying to figure out why I am so anxious. I don't understand this, where is this anxiety coming from?
>
> (Interviewee 1)

That is the one that I am most afraid of [Laughs]. I hate it. That is the one that has come up. I feel that I am questioning what this anxiety is. I haven't quite worked it out yet. It is a very difficult job being a mother and I don't think our society supports it. I don't think it is held up to be supported.

(Interviewee 2)

It is hard, especially if you are feeling anxious. The baby is just sitting there or he is asleep, if you know what I mean. Then he will get periods of crying and you don't know why. It is hard and very intense.

(Interviewee 3)

Then it started to escalate and I really didn't want to be left on my own with the baby. I was just really – very, very anxious.

(Interviewee 4)

This anxiety is not only at a cognitive level. This liminal anxiety sub-existed symbiotically with the 'unconscious suffering' that the mother needed to tolerate during this life-altering transition. This is a very difficult act to juggle and mothers are often overcome by a profound struggle within themselves. Maternal ambivalence is a direct consequence of this constant conflict with opposites in the liminal space. Out of this ambivalence, intense feelings erupt, such as anger, joy, love, shame, guilt, loneliness and sadness.

Most of the women interviewed felt or described the intensity of these feelings:

There is that sense of loss and sometimes you feel a bit bad about what you are just thinking.

(Interviewee 1)

Because how can you feel lonely if you have a child here? The loneliness is in my soul and that is important to me.

(Interviewee 2)

It is too much, yes. You just kind of didn't want to be responsible for somebody's life completely.

(Interviewee 3)

Specifically, I just feel much more deeply. It is like my experience of life is a lot more intense. There is more fear, love and joy.

(Interviewee 4)

This pattern of psychospiritual liminality has been understood as a form of psychological renewal and awakening of archetypal energy. It is a period where archetypes and symbols are quite significant for interpreting the profound depth of experience that mothers undergo in the transition to motherhood. Maternal ambivalence often arises because of the powerful archetype that is awakening in women at this liminal level: mother as both creator and destroyer (Parker 2005). All archetypal images necessarily have a dual nature, and the transpersonal psychologist, James Hillman (1990, 107), has noted this dichotomy within of the maternal archetype: 'You cannot have a good side without the other. The moment motherhood is constellated both sides are constellated. Nor is it possible to convert the negative into the positive'. In the coexistence of ambivalence, conflicts span and dualities in the new mother, new insights into truth and wisdom strive to be born. New ideas may emerge as barely explicit or 'half-hinted' consciousness (Damasio 1999). The unified and integrative self is often a glimpsed 'in-between' consciousness and unconsciousness. Some mothers have described it as learning to legislate for two states and to secure the border between them (Cusk 2001). The crisis that the transition to motherhood provokes and the journey into liminality has been described as a profound quest for wholeness and an authentic integrity for many women in the paradigm of the spiritual journey (Lombardi 2008).

Theme 2: embodiment and the conundrum of motherhood

The second theme that emerged in the pilot study of expanded consciousness through the transition to motherhood was embodiment. Women voiced the experience of a new connection with their bodies in relation to their maternal identities in numerous ways. The various subthemes revolved around pain, empowerment, change and sexuality.

Spirituality is intrinsically linked with the material body as well as with mind and spirit in human beings (McGuire 2003). In the second half of the twentieth century, a recovery of the integral unity of body-mind-spirit occurred. A spiritual sense of embodiment includes: body-based self-understanding, self-esteem manifested in the embrace of the body, self-acceptance of embodied identity and awareness of the bodily manifestation of affection and sexuality. The experience of embodied power is also at the core of our bodily health (Timmerman 2005). Women's bodies were historically viewed as unpredictable and chaotic. Indeed, the maternal body has been primarily governed, ordered and interpreted by religious institutions, as well as by the state and medical sciences (Kukla 2006).

Maternal embodiment inhabits a subjectivity that starts with the pregnant and lactating body. Imogen Tyler (2000, 290) described the unmapped, unthought-of and unthinkable of her pregnant body as: 'My body, my massive pregnant body.... Am I inappropriate? Monstrous? Am I obscene? Am I representable as an "I"? Am I?'.

The dichotomy of subject and object arises. Subjectivity resides in the liminal space of consciousness arising from the autonomous life processes in the lived body (Merleau-Ponty 1962). The relationship of subject and object in the self assumes multiple new forms, some of which cannot be articulated or even understood in 'higher cortex' mode but exist within body changes as embodied cognition (Langer 1948).

All of the women interviewed in this study spoke about the intense bodily connection with another and the unique feelings that this provokes:

> I passed him through between my legs. He was so slippy, I couldn't hold him. It was always so beautiful. This little baby has come out and you are connected to him. It is just so incredible. I held him in my arms for a while and then he fed.
>
> (Interviewee 1)

> When you see them, it is really exciting. It is certainly quite overwhelming. There is a protective … a fierce protection and a love, a fierce love but it is fiercer than I would have expected.
>
> (Interviewee 3)

> Yeah. I don't want to lose those feelings because they are so precious. They are just incredible. I could hold him then and. just the feeling and the connection.
>
> (Interviewee 4)

Maternal holding and connection not only includes the physical holding, but also a psychic holding relationship that provides ego-coverage for the infant. Thus, it has been argued that the mother and infant relationship is a chiasmic, embodied experience (Wynn 1997).

This embodied relationship challenges the woman's body and its boundaries as the relationship between the self and the infant is profoundly symbiotic. The boundaries between self and environment also become altered. In particular, the mother's kinetic experiences of the new-found clumsiness, slowness, delay, viscosity of the life in which she lives with her newborn child results in a range of heightened sensations that mothers very often report (Baraitser 2009). Women in this study also describe this kinetic experience:

> I wasn't able to have a shower. I couldn't speak to other people. I couldn't go to the loo. Having a shower was like luxury. Being able to text someone or check your emails or just be able to have a cup of tea [Laughs]. To finish having a cup of tea; I get to now. It took months before I was able to have a cup of tea and get to the bottom of the mug.
>
> (Interviewee 1)

> I always say you can tell how busy you are with babies by how many full cups of tea you have thrown down the sink because you never get a chance to drink them. There is always something happening. You don't really get a chance. I remember when I went back to work and I had a cup tea and just going – I am sitting here having a cup of tea and *I don't have to jump up* (researcher's emphasis).
>
> (Interviewee 3)

One recurrent topic that all mothers in this pilot study discussed was the relationship between maternal embodiment and sexuality. Research has shown that in the transition to motherhood, women encounter new restrictions on their sexuality (Friedman 1998). For most cultures, the desexualised mother is an important cultural construct in the discourse regarding what it is to be a 'woman' (Jones 2010). Rich (1976) asserted that the experience of motherhood is stereotypically characterised as a move in the woman towards an emphasis on femininity and nurturance, and a concomitant decreased emphasis on the woman as a sexual being. She believes that in a large cultural context, this characterisation is a pointing towards biological potential and also reveals the oppressive institutionalisation of motherhood (Rich 1976). There is a 'stand-back' in the sexuality of the woman in the liminal transition to motherhood. One woman in the study expressed this idea as follows:

> I think it is hilarious. I think it is separating something. In one way it's great because you are bringing sexuality into motherhood and you are not sexual anymore because you are a mother.
>
> (Interviewee 2)

> Yeah. There are two desires. There is desire about being desired, wanting to be desired and putting yourself out there well. Mothers are very much put into a box. You are not sexual anymore. I think you are definitely on a standby. I think this whole yummy mummy thing.
>
> (Interviewee 1)

Participants acknowledged the sexual transformation that had occurred while becoming a mother:

> For me sexuality as a mother has been completely deepened in me and it is intensified hugely which is amazing. I have moved from child to woman very much so and that is what it feels like. If I can connect with that and stay connected with that, it is lovely.
>
> (Interviewee 3)

> For me, it is about being a woman and what it means to be a woman and how I can express that and how I can embody that.
>
> (Interviewee 1)

Forming a deeper connection with sexual energy also alleviated symptoms of anxiety that one mother was experiencing:

> I feel disembodied most days. I was very breathless for the first few months. However, the more I connect in with my sexuality as a woman and what it means to me to be a woman, the less anxious I am.
>
> (Interviewee 1)

This account may indicate how an empowered sexual identity could have a transformative effect on anxiety, and the necessary challenge for the mother to differentiate inherited conflicted sexual feelings from the spiritual resource of her own creative energy. Research has shown how difficult a journey this may be, since culturally and historically, mothers have been displayed as un-desiring, non-sexual beings (O'Reilly 2010).

Adrienne Rich, has suggested that, in order for all women to have access to their innate potential for wisdom, they need to fully understand the power and powerlessness inscribed in the state of motherhood in patriarchal culture. One participant in this study made a link between her own power and the embodied experience of motherhood, as follows:

> I have realised how important being embodied is in my life because it gives me a sense of power, it is an empowerment.
>
> (Interviewee 1)

> Whereas, if I am conscious of my body, I am very much in the present and very much in the moment and I feel much more empowered.
>
> (Interviewee 3)

A lived consciousness of empowerment engenders feelings of transformation. Women in the study described this transformation in terms of acquiring a deeper consciousness, more inner growth, a great sense of mutual responsibility and an enriching sense of achievement in life.

Theme 3: philosophical liminal space and transformation

At the beginning of this chapter there was a description of how the liminal nature of birth requires the individual woman to incorporate herself into a new world. The new mother needs to transfer from the underworld of the birth experience into a ground-breaking adjustment and acceptance of her new self. The diverse emotions, desires, beliefs and values that were noted above as endemic to the crisis of motherhood are the fertile soil that will assist the growth of the mother's transformed self-awareness. This transformed self-awareness is essential for developing spiritual maturity (Wilber 2011). Women may require assistance in learning to reflect on the complexity of the conscious and unconscious thoughts and behaviours that are distinctive to the task of forming a maternal identity.

Self-reflection practices can be of assistance in increasing the introspection and inquiry that allow healing, self-acceptance and ultimately, the transformation which marks this stage in life (Siegel 2010). The mother starts accepting her responsibilities and reflecting on how these are changing her and her relationships. Most of the mothers in this study talked about feeling a sense of growing and maturing: 'It was a real milestone in your life. To become a parent, it does make you feel that bit more mature and older. I would never have thought about it before. I don't know if people see me differently' (Interviewee 4). Also, they reported the changes that motherhood made in their relationships with their partners:

> We would have had full blown arguments and we would have been shouting and you just can't do that. We have had to learn to negotiate differently, communicate differently and grow up.
>
> (Interviewee 1)

> Basically we have had to; it has been tough and very strenuous. We have had to grow up for one because you can't act out the way you used to act out in relationships. That has been incredibly trying. There is a huge amount of learning.
>
> (Interviewee 2)

The transformed mode of responsibility assumed in motherhood is closely linked to beliefs and core values that are important for the woman's sense of self identity (Looman 2003). A sense of achievement and reflective leadership may emerge for the woman in her newfound ability to manage difficult emotions.

Another study has shown that this reflective leadership is anchored in love (Scharmer 2009):

> There was such a rush of love. It is like the best drug ever. It was like wow! It is indescribable the feeling of achievement because we worked so hard at this.
>
> (Interviewee 1)

> I am not sure. I think lately and it has taken me years.... You do feel that your life is a little bit more complete. You do feel that it is a bit of an achievement. Like I said earlier, when people say: have you got any children? I am always really glad when I can say – yeah I do, I have one. Sometimes I wish I could say I have two or three.
>
> (Interviewee 4)

The development of self-awareness or self-consciousness through self-reflection along with the motivation and receptivity to engage with the unconscious processes that motherhood provokes will decide how far this transformation can be canalised in the life of the mother (Person 2002). Speaking of this transformative dynamic, mothers in this study recognised that the profound experience that they had gone through, when processed over time, had helped them to self-construct a transformed new self to engage the new realities of life:

> For me it means, I still have to remember who I am as opposed to as a mother and you know, that would be where I would fall down, I know myself so it is something that I wanted to be conscious of.
>
> (Interviewee 2)

Yeah. I can probably bring my own experience to it and my own depth of experience and what it means. I can bring my own spirituality to it and that is probably enough. However, I am looking more to connect. I want to help women to feel less alone.

(Interviewee 1)

To be honest with you, it took a good couple of years – it did take a good two years before; day by day I felt better and I started to feel more able.

(Interviewee 3)

This pilot study opens the question of what type of spiritual resources might further deepen the transition into motherhood. Such resources will cultivate the intrinsic spiritual are human capacities. Much research is needed to identify the different spiritual capacities that called forth in the maternal spiritual journey and for which appropriate supports might be developed.

This pilot study also shows the courage that the new mother needs in order to birth herself in the midst of the subjectivity blur which occurs in the experience of maternal liminality. Motherhood is a time in the life of women when encountering and struggling with the opposite dualities in the self is at its peak. Heraclitus wrote: 'Change is the constant conflict of opposites' and the 'universal logos of human nature' (Heraclitus 2003, 57–59).

There is a real potential for deep spiritual transformation in motherhood as there is also a potential for stagnation, depression and giving up. Ultimately, this pilot study has suggested that a more holistic awareness, an authentic self-acceptance and an expansion into new layers of empowering consciousness, can be spiritual gifts from the liminal space entered by the transition to motherhood. Deeper research into the conceptualisation of spirituality in the context of motherhood will assist women on the journey into motherhood to encounter the occasion as a moment of life-giving potential. This deeper conceptualisation is the focus on the next chapter, where the theory of spiritual intelligence is analysed.

Note

1 For the full definition of the word 'crisis', see: http://dictionary.cambridge.org/dictionary/english/crisis.

References

Akerjordet, K. 2010. 'Being in Charge – New Mothers' Perceptions of Reflective Leadership and Motherhood'. *Journal of Nursing Management* 18(4):409–417.

Baraitser, L. 2009. *Maternal Encounters. The Ethics of Interruption. Women and Psychology*. London: Routledge.

Barlow, C. 1997. 'Mothering as a Psychological Experience: A Grounded Theory Exploration'. *Canadian Journal of Counselling* 31(3):232–237.

Bragdon, E. 1993. *Helping People with Spiritual Problems*. Vermont, USA: Lightening Up Press.

Bragdon, E. 2013. *The Call of Spiritual Emergency*. San Francisco, USA: Harper and Row Publishers.

Carroll, R. 2003. 'At the Border between Chaos and Order'. In *Revolutionary Connections: Psychotherapy and Neuroscience*, edited by J. Corigall and H. Wilkinson, 191–211. New York: Karnac.

Cusk, R. 2001. *A Life's Work: On Becoming a Mother*. London: Fourth Estate Publisher.

Damasio, A. 1999. *The Feeling of What Happens: Body and Emotion in the Making of Consciousness*. New York: Harcourt Brace.

Darvill, R., Skirton, H., and Farrand, P. 2010. 'Psychological Factors that Impact on Women's Experiences of First-Time Mothers: A Qualitative Study of the Transition'. *Midwifery* 26:357–366.

Estes-Pinkola, C. 1996. *Women Who Run with the Wolves*. New York: Ballantine Books.

Friedman, A. 1998. 'Sexuality and Motherhood: Mutually Exclusive in Perception of Women'. *Sex Roles: A Journal of Research* 38(20):781–800.

Grof, S., and Grof, C. 1989. *Spiritual Emergency: When Personal Transformation Becomes a Crisis*. New York: TarcherPerigee.

Heraclitus. 2003. *Fragments*. London: Penguin Classics.

Hillman, J. 1990. 'The Bad Mother, an Archetypal Approach'. In *Fathers and Mothers*, edited by P. Berry, 107. Dallas, USA: Spring Publications.

Jones, R. 2010. 'Sexuality and Mothering'. In *Encyclopedia of Motherhood*, edited by A. O'Reilly, 1114–1116. Thousand Oaks, USA: Sage Publications.

Kukla, R. 2006. 'Introduction: Maternal Bodies'. *Hypatia* 21(1):7–9.

Lahood, G. 2007. 'Rumour of Angels and Heavenly Midwives: Anthropology of Transpersonal Events and Childbirth'. *Women and Birth* 20(7):3–10.

Langer, S. 1948. *Philosophy in a New Key: A Study in the Symbolism of Reason, Rite, and Art*. Oxford, UK: Oxford University Press.

Lombardi, N. 2008. 'Dancing in the Underworld: The Quest for Wholeness'. In *She Is Everywhere! Vol. 2: An Anthology of Writings in Womanist/Feminist Spirituality*, edited by A. Williams, 337–350. Lincoln, USA: iUniverse.

Looman, M. 2003. 'Reflective Leadership Strategic Planning from Heart and Soul'. *Consulting Psychology Journal Practice and Research* 55(4):215–221.

McGuire, M. 2003. 'Why Bodies Matter: A Sociological Reflection on Spirituality and Materiality'. *Spiritus: A Journal of Christian Spirituality* 3(1):1–18.

Merleau-Ponty, M. 1962. *The Phenomenology of Perception*. New York: Routledge and Kegan Paul.

Miller, J. 2004. *The Transcendent Function: Jung's Model of Psychological Growth through a Dialogue with the Unconscious*. New York: New York Press.

O'Reilly, A. 2010. 'Mothering, Sex and Sexuality'. *Encyclopedia of Motherhood*, 1115. London: Sage Publications.

Parker, R. 2005. *The Experience of Maternal Ambivalence. Torn in Two*. London: Virago Press.

Parratt, J., and Fahy, K. 2003. 'Trusting Enough to be out of Control: A Pilot Study of Women's Sense of Self during Childbirth'. *Australian Midwifery* 16(1):1522.

Person, E. 2002. *Feeling Strong. How Power Issues Affect Our Ability to Direct Our Own Lives*. New York: Harper Collins.

Rich, A. 1976. *Of a Woman Born: Motherhood as Experience and Institution*. New York: W. W. Norton & Company, Inc.

Scharmer, O. 2009. *Theory U Leading from the Future as it Emerges. Open Mind, Open Heart, Open Will. The Social Technology of Presencing*. San Francisco, USA: Berrett Koehler Publishers.

Searles, H. 1965. *Collected Works on Schizophrenia and Related Subjects*. London: Hogarth Press.

Siegel, D. 2010. *Mindsight, the New Science of Personal Transformation*. New York: Random House.

Steindl-Rast, D. 1985. *In Helping People with Spiritual Problems by E. Bragdon*. Vermont, USA: Lightening Up Press.

Timmerman, J. 2005. 'Body and Spirituality'. In *The New Westminster Dictionary of Christian Spirituality*, edited by P. Sheldrake, 153–155. London: SCM Press.

Turner, V. 1995. *The Ritual Process: Structure and Anti-Structure*. Piscataway, USA: Aldine Transaction.

Tyler, I. 2000. 'Reframing Pregnant Embodiment'. In *Transformation: Thinking through Feminism*, edited by A. Ahmed, J. Kilby, C. Lury, M. McNeil, and B. Skeggs, 288–301 London: Routledge.

Van Gennep, A. 2004. *The Rites of Passage*. London: Routledge.

Wilber, K. 1986. *Transformations of Consciousness: Conventional and Contemplative Perspectives on Development*. Boston, USA: Shambhala New Science Library.

Wilber, K. 2011. *Sex, Ecology, Spirituality: The Spirit of Evolution*. Boston, USA: Shambhala.

Wynn, F. 1997. 'The Embodied Chiasmic Relationship of Mother and Infant'. *Human Studies* 19:253–270.

5 Extending the psycho-spiritual paradigm

Spiritual intelligence theory

A key finding of the pilot study was the need to deepen the conceptualisation of spirituality for this type of study. In order to extend the psycho-spiritual paradigm, the theory of spiritual intelligence quotient (SQ) is examined. SQ and the different SQ capacities may assist in conceptualising unique maternal spiritual capacities that are called upon in the transition to motherhood.

Although understanding intelligence is a controversial issue among psychologists and other theorists, since the Harvard psychologist Howard Gardner proposed the theory of multiple intelligences (often abbreviated as MI theory), many questions have been posed regarding the understanding of 'intelligence'. Gardner describes intelligence not as one single entity, but as independent primary intelligences, including linguistic, logical-mathematical, musical, bodily-kinesthetic, spatial, intrapersonal, interpersonal, naturalist, moral and existential (Gardner 1983). This description opens an umbrella to questions such as: is intelligence only a representation of a physiological function of the brain neurons (Eysenck 1994) or is it a complex cognitive mechanism beyond biology? (Anderson 1992). If intelligence goes beyond cognitive processes, it can also be connected to other human domains, such as emotional content (Mayer and Salovey 1993). Other theorists have also defined intelligence as interlinked with personal virtues and moral conduct (Chiu et al. 1994; Sternberg and Kaufman 1998).

Intelligence is described as being made up of three parts: nature, nurture and results. Intelligence is an innate potential (nature), brought into form through practice (nurture) and results in adeptness or appropriately reasoned behaviour or choice (Wigglesworth 2012). If intelligence is mainly the human abilities (innate and acquired) to process knowledge, and how this knowledge guides and adapts people to an understanding of the world; spiritual intelligence can elucidate unique spiritual capacities (innate/acquired) that human beings use in this adaptation.

Analysing different theorists on Spiritual Intelligence and their spiritual capacities may open a door on how those capacities are interlinked with the current research on the lived experience of motherhood studies.

Spiritual intelligence theory

The term 'spiritual intelligence' was coined by Danah Zohar when she intro-duced the idea in 1997. In her book (1997), she proposed that spiritual intelli-gence is at the top of a hierarchy representing the brain's integrative processes (as meaning-making values). She believed that intelligence quotient (IQ), emo-tional quotient (EQ) and spiritual quotient (SQ) correspond to three distinct neural arrangements in the brain. Emotional intelligence is behind reflecting the brain's associative processes and at the bottom of the hierarchy are the rational intelligences (Zohar 2001). Zohar's model reflected a holistic approach to human intelligence as it integrated the physical, mental, emotional and spiritual. She outlined eight components in SQ: (1) a high degree of self-awareness; (2) having the capacity of flexibility (active and spontaneous adaptation); (3) having the capacity of dealing with pain and its development; (4) the tendency to ask ques-tions of why or how, and searching for key answers; (5) being inspired by imagi-nation and values; (6) the tendency to see the links between different things (being holistic); (7) unwillingness to injure; and (8) getting away from the context that facilitates unconventional activity (Zohar and Marshall 2001).

Zohar's model suggested that emotional intelligence is the most closely linked to spiritual intelligence, but she also hypothesised the notion of the exist-ence of a connection between intelligences:

> It provides a context for our actions, as well as the way we assess whether one course of action or one life-path is more meaningful than another. SQ is the necessary foundation for the effective functioning of both IQ and EQ. It is our ultimate intelligence.
>
> (Zohar and Marshall 2001, 3)

Following Zohar's studies at the beginning of the 2000s, other theorists start questioning claims of spirituality as a distinct type of human capability. Robert Emmons (2000, 4) also explored spirituality as a form of intelligence and he defined spirituality as: 'the adaptive use of spiritual information to facilitate everyday problem solving and goal attainment'.

He asserted that similar to consciousness, SQ is an individual's capacity to have a sense of sacredness, virtue and the awareness that everything is intercon-nected in the universe. He outlines five components of SQ: (1) the capacity for transcendence; (2) the ability to enter into heightened spiritual states of con-sciousness; (3) the ability to invest everyday activities, events and relationships with a sense of the sacred; (4) the ability to utilise spiritual resources to solve problems in living; and (5) the capacity to engage in virtuous behaviour (to show forgiveness, to express gratitude, to be humble, to display compassion) (Emmons 2000).

Similarly, Professor and psychologist, Kathleen D. Noble, stated that spiritual intelligence integrates the qualities of flexibility and emotional resilience (that may arise out of spiritual experiences), which play a role in psychological health and behaviour. She agrees with Emmons's main components of SQ, but added two more capacities related to consciousness (Noble 2001):

1   Conscious recognition in which physical reality is formulated continuously within a larger multi-dimensional reality that we deal with it consciously or unconsciously.
2   Conscious pursuit of psychological health not only for ourselves but for all of society.

She also believed that SQ is an innate human potential and that SQ is interconnected with EQ.

Psychologist, Frances Vaughan, also understands SQ as an insight that people have about themselves and by which they regulate their own emotions. She believes that SQ is concerned with the inner life of mind and spirit and its relationship to being in the world (Vaughan 2002). As with previous theorists discussed above, Vaughan connects SQ intimately with EQ. She maintains that SQ is more than an individual mental ability. It connects the personal to the transpersonal and the self to spirit. SQ goes beyond conventional psychological development.

Like emotion, spiritual intelligence calls for multiple ways of knowing and has varying degrees of depth and expression. Vaughan asserts that everyone has the potential for developing spiritual intelligence, just as everyone has a capacity for intuition, thinking, sensing and feeling (Vaughan 1979). For Vaughan, SQ depends at least on three distinct ways of knowing: sensory, rational and contemplative. These three ways of knowing appear to be an integral part of the spiritual intelligence. Contemplative practices such as meditation, prayer or yoga seem particularly relevant for refining spiritual intelligence, and such practises engage those three ways of knowing (Vaughan 2002). She outlines eight capacities of SQ: openness, integrity, humility, kindness, generosity, tolerance and resistance and desire to meet others' needs. These capacities will enhance the cultivation of authenticity and self-awareness (Vaughan 2002).

Spiritual intelligence, as explained by most of the theorists above, not only involves existential capacities, but exists as a set of mental abilities that are distinct from behavioural traits and experiences (King and DeCicco 2009). Researcher on spiritual intelligence, David King (2008, 69) defines SQ as: 'The awareness, integration, and adaptive application of the nonmaterial and transcendent aspects of one's existence leading to such outcomes as deep existential reflection, enhancement of meaning, recognition of a transcendent self, and mastery of spiritual states'. King outlines four components of SQ: critical existential thinking, personal meaning production, transcendental awareness and conscious state expansion. He argues that aspects of cognition are inherent in the discussion of existential thinking, existential contemplation and existential reasoning. In his book, *Rethinking Claims of Spiritual Intelligence: A Definition, Model and Measure*, King tried to deal directly with the main criticism of SQ formulated by leading intelligence theorists Gardner and Mayer. These theorists are still not satisfied with the term 'intelligence': indeed, Mayer actually prefers to refer it as 'spiritual consciousness' (Mayer 2000). They believe that without cognition, the term intelligence cannot be used. This is the reason why Gardner (1983) did not include SI in his multiple intelligence theory, because it was difficult to quantify with scientific criteria.

King has also investigated the relationship between spiritual and emotional intelligence in the only study to date (King *et al.* 2012). He believes that examining spiritual and emotional intelligence together is a critical step in the theoretical and statistical investigation of this emerging construct. He has also created the first Spiritual Intelligence Self-Report Inventory instrument (SISRI-24) to measure SQ.[1] The first component of SQ that King proposes (the spiritual capacity of critical thinking) requires cognition and emotions. The type of cognitive-emotional thinking outlined by King is actively and skilfully conceptualising, applying, analysing and synthesising and evaluating information gathered by observation, experience, reflection, reasoning or communication. Critical thinking is self-directed, self-disciplined, self-monitored and self-corrective thinking (Scriven and Paul 2013).

Most spiritual and wisdom traditions cultivate a universal set of existential qualities that are adaptive. A study by researcher, Yosi Amram, showed that spiritual intelligence can be applied in every moment of daily life so as to experience the greater meaning and wellbeing facilitated by practising qualities such as mindfulness, presence and compassion, even in the face of pain and suffering (Amram 2007a). In this study, Amram outlines seven capacities in SQ that are nearly universal across the great wisdom traditions of Buddhism, Christianity, Hinduism, Islam, Judaism, Shamanism, Taoism and Yoga. These are: (1) internal knowledge; (2) deep intuition; (3) self-awareness, integrating with nature and the universe; (4) the ability to solve problems, (5) inner guidance and using sublimation methods such as intuition; (6) acceptance and love of truth; and (7) a holistic view in order to see the interconnections among things (Amram 2009).

As with any human intelligence, the full understanding, expression and integration of these capacities will contribute to 'living authentically the full possibilities of being human' (Anastoos 1998). In 'living authentically', Vaughan asserts that with commitment and integrity, this path can lead from the bondage of unconsciousness to spiritual freedom, from fear and defensiveness to love and compassion and from ignorance and confusion to wisdom and understanding (Vaughan 2002). Compassion is at the core of theorist Cindy Wigglesworth's (2004, 4) definition of spiritual intelligence: 'The ability to behave with compassion and wisdom while maintaining inner and outer peace (equanimity) regardless of the circumstances'.

Spiritual intelligence enables one to recognise the value of qualities such as compassion in others, as well as within oneself. At the moment, ongoing studies on the relationship between spiritual intelligence and health and workplace and psychological development are being researched (Azizi and Zamaniyan 2013; Hosseini *et al.* 2010; King *et al.* 2012; Koohbanani *et al.* 2013; Singh and Sinha

Table 5.1 Definitions of spiritual intelligence

Author/year	Definition of spiritual intelligence
Zohar and Marshal (2001, 4)	'A context for our actions, as well as the way we assess whether one course of action or one life-path is more meaningful than another. SQ is the necessary foundation for the effective functioning of both IQ and EQ. It is our ultimate intelligence'.[1]
Emmons (2000, 4)	'The adaptive use of spiritual information to facilitate everyday problem solving and goal attainment'.
Noble (2000, 2)	'An innate human potential'.
Vaughan (2002, 3)	'Spiritual intelligence is concerned with the inner life of mind and spirit and its relationship to being in the world'.
King and DeCicco (2009, 69)	'Spiritual intelligence contributes to the awareness, integration, and adaptive application of the nonmaterial and transcendent aspects of one's existence'.
Amram (2007a, 1)	'Spiritual intelligence is defined as the as the ability to apply and embody spiritual resources and qualities to enhance daily functioning and wellbeing'.
Wigglesworth (2002–2004, 4)	'The ability to behave with Compassion and Wisdom while maintaining inner and outer peace (equanimity) regardless of the circumstances'.

Note
1 SQ, spiritual intelligence quotient; IQ, intelligence quotient; EQ, emotional quotient.

2013; Suan Chin *et al.* 2011). SQ is not only about individual self-development but it transcends into service for others. Wigglesworth has created a competency-based language that helps people to think about what they want in their own spiritual development. She believes that SQ will not only benefit individuals, but their families, communities and the companies they work for. This faith-neutral language of competencies will make SQ acceptable for discussion in the workplace. Wigglesworth's SQ capacities/skills create a more meaningful work, improved products and services and ensure responsible corporate behaviour (Wigglesworth 2004).

Table 5.1 shows the main definitions of spiritual intelligence

Spiritual capacities

By comparing the different definitions outlined in Table 5.1, many describing factors began to converge, diver and overlap. Intelligence has been defined as being composed of three parts: nature, nurture and results in adeptness (Wigglesworth 2012). One definition considers spiritual intelligence as an innate capacity, thus, part of human nature and congenital (Noble 2001). Most of the definitions related in Table 5.1 are more interested in describing the nurture part of spiritual intelligence through the process of adaptation (Emmons 2000; King 2008) and the diverse practices used in the process (Amram 2007a; 2007b; King 2008; Wigglesworth 2012; Zohar and Marshall 2001). Some authors overlap in the unique spiritual capacities that are needed in order to achieve everyday adaptation to life. Both Zohar and Marshall (2001) and Amram (2007b) highlight the search of a life-path that can deepen every day experiences to greater meaning. Amram (2007b) and Wigglesworth (2012) mention quality of compassion as necessary for wellbeing and peace in facing pain and suffering. Other spiritual capacities singled out in the definitions are: mindfulness and presence (Amram 2007a), awareness and transcendent aspects (King 2008) and wisdom (Wigglesworth 2012). Overall, the definitions above describe spiritual intelligence as innate, and also as nurture (the need to practice and apply spiritual capacities with the goal of adapting to everyday living and reducing the suffering of one's existence). Every author also further develops unique spiritual capacities through his/her own research on spiritual intelligence. These spiritual capacities are listed in Table 5.2.

In Table 5.2, each capacity is highlighted by a different symbol (*, †, ‡, ¶ and #). If a capacity appears in three authors or more, it is singled out and further analysed. Five main spiritual capacities emerged from Table 5.2: (1) personal meaning production (*); (2) consciousness/awareness (†); (3) self-reflection/ reflexivity (‡); (4) creativity (¶); and (5) transpersonal orientation (#). Below are the capacities that appear in more than in three authors.

Table 5.2 Listing of spiritual capacities, by author

Author/year	Spiritual capacities[1]
Zohar and Marshal (2001, 15)	1 A high degree of self-awareness.†
	2 Having the capacity of flexibility (active and spontaneous adaptation).‡
	3 Having the capacity of dealing with pains and its development.*
	4 Tend to ask questions of why or how, and search for key answers.*
	5 Getting inspire of the imaginations and values.¶
	6 The tendency to see the links between different things (being holistic).*
	7 Unwillingness to injure.‡
	8 Getting away from the context that facilitates unconventional activity.¶
Emmons (2000, 10)	1 The capacity for transcendence (going beyond physical and material world and making them excellent).#
	1 The ability to enter into heightened spiritual states of consciousness.†
	2 The ability to invest everyday activities, events, and relationships with a sense of the sacred.¶
	4 The ability to utilise spiritual resources to solve problems in living.#
	5 The capacity to be virtuous and to engage in virtuous behaviour (generosity, gratefulness, humility and kindness).‡

Noble (2001, 3)	Emmons' capacities and two more added: 1 Conscious recognition that physical reality is embedded within a larger, multidimensional reality.† 2 Conscious pursuit (the choice to develop psychospiritual awareness in order to promote the health of both the individual and the global community).†
Vaughan (2002, 8)	1 Openness.‡ 2 Integrity.¶ 3 Humility.‡ 4 Kindness.‡ 5 Generosity.¶ 6 Tolerance.‡ 7 Resistance.‡ 8 Desire to meet other needs.*
King and DeCicco (2009, 69–71)	1 Critical existential thinking.‡ 2 Personal meaning production.* 3 Transcendental awareness.† 4 Conscious state expansion.†
Amram (2009, 17)	1 Internal knowledge.‡ 2 Deep intuition.‡ 3 Self-awareness and integrating with nature and the universe.† 4 Ability to solving problems.* 5 Inner guidance and using sublimation methods such as intuition to solve problems.* 6 Acceptance and love of truth.‡ 7 Holistic view in order to see the interconnections among things, etc.# (consciousness,† grace, meaning,* transcendence,# truth, peaceful surrender to self‡ and inner-directedness‡)
Wigglesworth (2003, 10)	1 Higher self/ego self-awareness (awareness of own worldview, awareness of life purpose (mission), awareness of values hierarchy, complexity of inner thought, awareness of ego self/higher self).† 2 Universal awareness† (awareness of interconnectedness of all life, awareness of worldviews of others, breadth of time perception, awareness of limitations/power of human perception, awareness of spiritual laws, experience of transcendent oneness).# 3 Higher self/ego self-mastery (commitment to spiritual growth, keeping higher self in charge, living your purpose and values, sustaining your faith, seeking guidance from spirit).¶ 4 Social mastery/spiritual presence (wise and effective spiritual teacher/mentor, wise and effective change agent, making compassionate and wise decisions, calming/healing presence and being aligned with the ebb/flow of life).¶

Note

1 Spiritual capacities are coded with symbols to facilitate the review (personal meaning production (*); consciousness/awareness (†); self-reflection/reflexivity (‡); creativity (¶); and transpersonal orientation (#)).

Personal meaning production (*)

This capacity has been explored as a component of spiritual intelligence by most of theorists and more specifically by Zohar (2001), King (2008; 2010) and Amram (2007a). Once a crucial life experience happens, the ability to produce personal meaning and purpose is extremely adaptive. Research has shown how meaning production impacts on social roles, relationships, basic needs, personal growth, work, achievement and even dreams (Jung 1960; Thompson 1992; Wong 1989). Sources of meaning are limitless. Crisis is also related to meaning production since it challenges our capacity to make sense of suffering and pain.

This capacity is crucially related to human survival. Victor Frankl described existential crisis as 'the frustration of the will to meaning' (Frankl 1969). Coping with many stressors will be validated and alleviated if the individual is capable of constructing meaning (Parks 1998). Meaning plays a significant role in both the maintenance of hope and prevention of anxiety and depression (Mascaro and Rosen 2005). King (2008) revealed by his research that people vary in terms of their capacity to derive or create meaning and purpose (Reker and Chamberlain 2000; Zika and Chamberlain 1992) and that there is little doubt as to the cognitive operations which enable one to construct meaning (Meddin 1998; Wong 1989). Meaning is frequently included in the definitions of spirituality (Wink and Dillon 2002, Worthington and Sandage 2001), so its inclusion in SQ is both natural and necessary (King 2008). Meaning-making capacity does not work in isolation, but in relation to others. It is important to note that SQ is not an adaptive anthropological concept that has served only the individual, but it must expand into service of the collective human race. Amram (2009) explores meaning capacity as experiencing significance in daily activities through a sense of purpose and a call for service, including in the face of pain and suffering. Zohar (2001) sees SQ as emerging from our most basic and primary need for and experience of deep meaning in life.

Consciousness/awareness (†)

Consciousness is probably the one capacity that is included in multiple studies in spirituality. Most theorists include consciousness in their list of capacities characteristic to SQ (see Table 5.2). Leading intelligence theorist, John Mayer, described spiritual intelligence as 'heightened consciousness' and 'structuring consciousness', so problems are seen in the context of life's ultimate concerns. Consciousness is to be aware of emotion, motivation and cognition and consequently is quite intrinsically interlinked with these three systems in human beings (Mayer 2000). Consciousness is defined (Rao 2002, 15) as: 'A state of self-awareness in which there is a reflexive relationship between the phenomena of experience and the experiencing person'.

Vaughan explains SQ as a capacity for deep understanding of existential questions and insight into multiple levels of consciousness (Vaughan 2002). Spiritual intelligence is a way of 'being and experiencing' and is focused on consciousness (Elkins *et al.* 1988). Emmons' (2000) and Noble's (2001) research into SQ suggests that in order for lived experiences to evolve into SQ, an individual's conscious awareness needs to help him or her to an understanding of the meaning of those experiences and in integrating them mindfully into the totality of his or her personal and community life. SQ is crucial in this process, as these experiences can have a profound effect biologically, psychologically, intellectually and interpersonally – not always positive (Green and Noble 2010). The concept of conscious awareness is very important in a transition where new experiences are trying to create meaning for an individual's identity and self. Noble asserts that individuals must learn to tolerate uncertainty and paradox to be able to explore the larger phenomena of reality. SQ is necessary to tolerate difficult feelings such as confusion and uncertainty. King recognises the ability to move beyond self-centred consciousness, to see things with a considerable measure of freedom from biological and social conditioning (King *et al.* 2012).

The recognition and ongoing awareness of a transcendent self is a key component of becoming conscious. Other components, such as in-depth perception and discernment, are part of conscious awareness in the individual. These components describe cognitive abilities of awareness that exist outside of ordinary consciousness, including holism and transcendent aspects of the self and others. Wigglesworth (2012) described two types of self-awareness: the ego self-awareness and the universal awareness that interconnects all life together. The capacity of conscious awareness overlaps with most SQ capacities, as it seems to be the core from which the others operate by producing a different type of knowledge. Amram's research on SQ shows that consciousness capacity develops a self-knowledge that he calls a 'trans-rational knowing'. This is a knowledge that transcends rationality through synthesis of paradoxes and using various states/modes of consciousness as meditation, prayer, silence, intuition, and dreams (Amram 2007a).

Self-reflection/reflexivity (‡)

Self-reflection is described as the bridge and the intermediary between self-awareness and self-transformation. This spiritual capacity is the one that triggers the deep responses of change and adaptation after any challenging experience happens. Reflection also provides the ability to revise the 'meaning structures' (Taylor 2000). Most theorists have researched this capacity within their own framework. Zohar's capacity of flexibility (active and spontaneous adaptation) and Vaughan's capacities of openness, humility and tolerance are related to reflective power (2002). Self-reflection will help to increase introspection and inquiry and also allow an openness to the experience in terms of healing, self-acceptance and ultimately, transformation (Zohar and Marshall 2001). This reflection power is to see the 'why' and 'what if' in addition to 'what' and 'how'. Another quality of this deep reflection is its critical orientation to one's own and others' understanding (Kim 2004). Noble explains it as an acceptance of all parts of ourselves, both the good and the bad, and a becoming more compassionate and tolerant of individual differences. This capacity is extremely important in maternal ambivalence. If self-reflection manages to integrate experiences into the person's life, it can lead to a greater understanding and ability to endure adversity, confusion, conflicting feelings, self-destructives attitudes and behaviours (Green and Noble 2010).

For Vaughan, self-reflection is the ability to recognise and utilise inner resources such as intuition, particularly empathy and humility. In her book, *Awakening Intuition*, she writes (1979, 181): 'The stabilization of intuitive insights, and their usefulness to humanity, are subsequently determined by careful, logical examination and validation, but the original vision or insight is intuitive'. King's research on SQ showed that many individuals display a heightened or above average sense of intuition in the SISRI instrument he developed. His SQ capacity on critical existential thinking is believed to be generated by reflection, experiencing and reasoning (King and DeCicco 2009). Self-reflection has the ability to create knowledge in the individual through the synthesis of paradoxes and transcending rationality. Amram's SQ capacity on trans-rational knowing is intimately embedded in the capacity of reflection of the individual (Amram 2007a; 2007b). This reflective inner knowledge is crucial in the development of important qualities in SQ such as: kindness, self-forgiveness, self-compassion and self-acceptance.

Creativity (¶)

In a truly transformative experience, the power of creativity will frequently be opened. Wigglesworth (2012) has created 21 SQ abilities which can help in becoming a spiritual conscious leader in business. SQ abilities have been proven paramount in the leadership success in the twenty-first century. Creative capacities are described as discovering one's personal gifts and strengths, use of imagination or even the bringing of a fresh perspective to situations in one's life (Johnson 2011). Zohar's model can be used to explain the relationship between creativity and spiritual intelligence, in which a necessary precondition for spontaneity, initiative and creativity is required (Zohar and Marshall 2001). Creativity, spontaneity and vision are used to deal with existential problems. According to Zohar and Marshall, individuals who fully develop their creativity have a better possibility of coping with despair, pain, suffering and loss.

There is a meaningful relationship between spiritual intelligence and creativity in people. The creative is the power of the imagination to transform. This capacity is a truly spiritual experience and it is commonly associated with feelings of clarity, connection, opening and energy (Vaughan 2002). Several dimensions of intelligence have a certain effect on creating creativity in people (Amram 2005). Creativity has been linked with the liberation from fears and a manifestation of courage (Amram 2007a). Campbell, in writing about the hero's journey, referred to motherhood as: 'creation, the source of life and nourishment is now within the mother herself' (Campbell 2012).

The creative capacity will depend in great measure on the above capacities already mentioned, such as the development of self-awareness, consciousness and self-reflection, along with the motivation and receptivity to unconscious processes; and it will decide how far any transformation will be canalised into a creative expression (Person 2002).

Transpersonal orientation: transcendence/transcendental (#)

As most theorists have articulated, the transpersonal dimension is included in the study of SQ (Emmons 2000; Noble 1987; 2000; 2001). Spirituality is concerned with the study of humanity's deepest potential and the recognition, under-standing and realisation of spiritual and transcendent states of consciousness (Lajoie and Shapiro 1992).

The experiences encompassed by this concept are complex phenomena with cognitive, emotional, biological, religious and cultural components. They are extremely diverse and have been reported in every culture and era. Archetypi-cally, when a rite of passage happens, the person is not the same after the experi-ence, either physically or psychically. It provokes a fundamental change in consciousness. Jung believed that these experiences provoke a breakdown in the psyche which can lead to psychosis, unless the materials can be translated into communicable symbols, archetypes or states that can canalise these powers into consciousness (Jung 1967). Pregnancy, birth and the transition to motherhood have been found to create conditions that they are ritualistic in nature and some-times visionary states have emerged (Davis-Floyd 1992; Klassen 2001; Lahood 2006). Such experiences arrive in a plethora of ways: between individuals and the sacred, extrasensory perceptions, dreams and altered states of consciousness, meditation, listening to music, being in nature and attending religious services. These experiences arise spontaneously, while others are the result of committed contemplative practice (Noble 2000; 2001). Noble's and Emmons' research delineated the capacity for transcendence in SQ as one of the key factors in spir-itual intelligence. Studies have shown that positive psychological wellbeing may be related to transcendent experiences. Transcendence beliefs are associated with greater proficiency in the acquisition and use of acquired knowledge, as well as better psychological abilities (Lukey and Baruss 2004). The capacity to tran-scendent dimensions of the self what – Maslow called 'self-actualization' – is the ability to sense a spiritual dimension of life, engaging other capacities such as self-reflection, awareness and consciousness (Wolman 2001). Building on Maslow's work, the capacity to self-transcend has been described as a process of transcendent-actualisation, which is a self-realisation founded on an awareness and experience of a spiritual centre in the individual (Hamel *et al.* 2003). The transpersonal capacity is described as individuals who 'move beyond the bound-aries of their personal limitations by integrating individual goals with larger ones, such as the welfare of the family, the community, humanity, the planet, or the cosmos' (Csikszentmihalyi 1994, 219). Amram also understood this capacity as going beyond oneself and attachment to the greater whole (Amram 2005). It is an interrelated wholeness incorporating a holistic system's standpoint and fostering human relationships by appreciating, sympathy and I-Thou orientation (Amram 2009).

The five capacities outlined above show that spiritual intelligence involves a kind of adaptability and problem-solving behaviour which involves the highest levels of growth in different cognitive, ethical, emotional and interpersonal fields. Emotional intelligence is the capacity to understand our own emotions, but spiritual intelligence is the ability to appreciate the meaning and the existential context of those emotions. Modernity repressed the 'higher levels of spiritual intelligence' due to understanding spirituality erroneously as a form of pre-modern religious repressions. Postmodernism has blamed the rational for such repression and has protected spirituality from excessive rationality and reductionist intelligence theory.

By singling out spiritual capacities from the theory of spiritual intelligence, a new relationship can be linked with such capacities and the current literature on the transition to motherhood.

In Part III of this book, spirituality and motherhood are conceptualised by research in the maternal literature. Articles on spirituality and motherhood are investigated in the light of these five capacities or any others that may emerge to further extend unique maternal spiritual capacities that can assist mothers in their transition.

Note

1 The SISRI-24 document can be found online here: www.davidbking.net/spiritual intelligence/sisri-24.pdf.

References

Amram, Y. 2005. *The Seven Development and Preliminary Validation of the Integrated Spiritual Intelligence Scale (ISIS) Paper*. www.Geocities. Cam/isisfindings/.

Amram, Y. 2007a. *The Seven Dimensions of Spiritual Intelligence: An Ecumenical Grounded Theory*. Paper presented at the 115th annual conference of the American Psychological Association, San Francisco, USA, August 2007.

Amram, Y. 2007b. *What is Spiritual Intelligences? An Ecumenical, Grounded Theory*. Working paper of the Institute of Transpersonal Psychology, Palo Alto, USA.

Amram, Y. 2009. *The Contribution of Emotional and Spiritual Intelligences to Effective Business Leadership*. PhD Diss., Institute of Transpersonal Psychology, Palo Alto, CA, USA.

Anastoos, C. 1998. 'Humanistic Psychology and Ecopsychology'. *The Humanistic Psychologist* 26:34.

Anderson, M. 1992. *Intellignce and Development: A Cognitive Theory*. Cambridge, USA: Blackwell.

Azizi, M., and Zamaniyan, M. 2013. 'The Relationship between Spiritual Intelligence and Vocabulary Learning Strategies in EFL Learners'. *Theory and Practice in Language Studies* 3(5):852–858.

Campbell, J. 2012. *The Hero with a Thousand Faces. The Collected Works of Joseph Campbell*. Novato, USA: New World Library.

Chiu, C., Hong, Y., and Dweck, C. 1994. 'Toward an Integrative Model of Personality and Intelligence: A General Framework and Some Preliminary Steps'. In *Personality and Intelligence*, edited by R. Sternberg and P. Ruzgis, 104–134. Cambridge, UK: Cambridge University Press.

Csikszentmihalyi, M. 1994. *The Evolving Self: A Psychology for the Third Millennium*. New York: Harper Perennial Press.

Davis-Floyd, R. 1992. *Birth as an American Rite of Passage*. Oakland, USA: University of California Press.

Elkins, D., Hedstrom, J., Hughes, L., Leaf, A., and Saunders, C. 1988. 'Toward a Humanistic-Phenomenological Spirituality'. *Journal of Humanistic Psychology* 28(4):5–18.

Emmons, R. 2000. 'Is Spirituality an Intelligence? Motivation, Cognition and the Psychology of Ultimate Concern'. *The International Journal for the Psychology of Religion* 10:3–26.

Eysenck, M. 1994. *Individual Differences. Normal and Abnormal*. Oxon, UK: Psychology Press.

Frankl, V. 1969. *The Will to Meaning*. New York: New American Library.

Gardner, H. 1983. *Frames of Mind: The Theory of Multiple Intelligences*. New York: Basic Books.

Green, W., and Noble, K. 2010. 'Fostering Spiritual Intelligence: Undergraduates' Growth in a Course about Consciousness'. *Advanced Development Journal* 12:26–48.

Hamel, S., Leclerc, G., and Lefrançois, R. 2003. 'A Psychological Outlook on the Concept of Transcendent Actualization'. *The International Journal for the Psychology of Religion* 13:3–15.

Hosseini, M., Elias, H., Krauss, S., and Aishah, S. 2010. 'A Review Study on Spiritual Intelligence, Adolescence and Spiritual Intelligence: Factors that May Contribute to Individual Differences in Spiritual Intelligence, and the Related Theories'. *International Journal of Psychological Studies* 2(2):179–188.

Johnson, P. 2011. 'An Atlantic Genealogy of "Spirit Possession"'. *Comparative Studies in Society and History* 53:393–425.

Jung, C. 1960. *The Structure and Dynamics of the Psyche*. London: Routledge.

Jung, C. 1967. 'Symbols of Transformation (1912)'. In *Collected Works, Volume 5*, translated by R. F. C. Hull. Princeton, USA: Princeton University Press.

Kim, Y. 2004. 'Spirituality and Affect: A Function of Changes in Religious Affiliation'. *Journal of Family Psychology* 13(3):17–25.

King, D. 2008. *Rethinking Claims of Spiritual Intelligence: A Definition, Model, & Measure*. Ontario, Canada: Trent University Press.

King, D. 2010. 'Personal Meaning Production as a Component of Spiritual Intelligence'. *International Journal of Existential Psychology and Psychotherapy* 3(1):1–5.

King, D., and DeCicco, T. 2009. 'A Viable Model and Self-Report Measure of Spiritual Intelligence'. *International Journal of Transpersonal Studies* 28:68–85.

King, D., Mara, C., and DeCicco, T. 2012. 'Connecting the Spiritual and Emotional Intelligences: Confirming an Intelligence Criterion and Assessing the Role of Empathy'. *International Journal of Transpersonal Studies* 31:11–20.

Klassen, P. 2001. *Blessed Events: Religion and the Home Birth Movement in America*. Princeton, USA and Oxford, UK: Princeton University.

Koohbanani, E., Dastjerdi, B., Vahidi, T., and Ghani, M. 2013. 'The Relationship between Spiritual Intelligence and Emotional Intelligence with Life Satisfaction among Birjand Gifted Female High School Students'. *Social and Behavioral Sciences* 84:314–320.

Lahood, G. 2006. 'Skulls at the Banquet: Near Birth as Nearing Death'. *Journal of Transpersonal Psychology* 38(1):1–24.

Lajoie, D., and Shapiro, S. 1992. 'Definitions of Transpersonal Psychology: The First Twenty-three Years'. *Journal of Transpersonal Psychology* 24(1):79–98.

Lukey, N., and Baruss, I. 2004. 'Intelligence Correlates of Transcendent Beliefs: A Preliminary Study'. *Imagination, Cognition, and Personality* 24(3):259–270.

Mascaro, N., and Rosen, D. 2005. 'Existential Meaning's Role in the Enhancement of Hope and Prevention of Depressive Symptoms'. *Journal of Personality* 73:985–1014.

Mayer, J. D. 2000. 'Spiritual Intelligence or Spiritual Consciousness?'. *The International Journal for the Psychology of Religion* 10(1):47–56.

Mayer, J. D., and Salovey, P. 1993. 'The Intelligence of Emotional Intelligence'. *Intelligence* 17: 433–442.

Meddin, J. 1998. 'Dimensions of Spiritual Meaning and Well-Being in the Lives of Ten Older Australians'. *International Journal of Aging and Human Development* 47:163–175.

Noble, K. 1987. 'Psychological Health and the Experience of Transcendence'. *The Counseling Psychologist* 15:601–614.

Noble, K. 2000. 'Spiritual Intelligence: A New Frame of Mind'. *Advanced Development* 9:1–29.

Noble, K. 2001. *Riding the Windhorse: Spiritual Intelligence and the Growth of the Self.* Cresskill, USA: Hampton Press.

Parks, C. 1998. 'Coping with Loss'. *British Medical Journal* 316:1521–1524.

Person, E. 2002. *Feeling Strong. How Power Issues Affect Our Ability to Direct Our Own Lives.* New York: Harper Collins.

Rao, K. 2002. 'What Is It Like to Be Conscious?'. In *Consciousness Studies. Cross Cultural Perspectives*, edited by the International Society for Sciences and Religion. ISSR Library. Jefferson, USA: McFarland and Company, Inc. Publishers.

Reker, G., and Chamberlain, K. eds 2000. *Exploring Existential Meaning: Optimizing Human Development across the Life Span.* Thousand Oaks, USA: SAGE.

Scriven, M., and Paul, R. 2013. *Defining Critical Thinking. Foundation for Critical Thinking.* www.criticalthinking.org/pages/defining-critical-thinking/410.

Singh, M., and Sinha, J. 2013. 'Impact of Spiritual Intelligence on Quality of Life'. *International Journal of Scientific and Research Publications* 3(5):1–5.

Sternberg, R., and Kaufman, J. 1998. 'Human Abilities'. *Annual Review of Psychology* 49: 479–502.

Suan Chin, S., Anantharaman, R., and Kin Tong, D. 2011. 'The Roles of Emotional Intelligence and Spiritual Intelligence at the Workplace'. *Journal of Human Resources Management Research* 2011:9.

Taylor, B. 2000. Deep Ecology and its Social Philosophy: A Critique'. In *Beneath the Surface: Critical Essays on Deep Ecology*, edited by E. Katz, A. Light, and D. Rothenberg, 269–299. Cambridge, USA: MIT Press.

Thompson, P. 1992. '"I Don't Feel Old": Subjective Ageing and the Search for Meaning in Later Life'. *Ageing and Society* 12:23–47.

Vaughan, F. 1979. *Awakening Intuition.* New York: Doubleday/Anchor.

Vaughan, F. 2002. 'What is Spiritual Intelligence?'. *Journal of Humanistic Psychology* 42(2):3, 16–33.

Wigglesworth, C. 2002–2004. *Spiritual Intelligence and Why It Matters.* Missoula, USA: Conscious Pursuits Inc.

Wigglesworth, C. 2003. *Spiritual Intelligence: What Is It? How Can We Measure It? Why Would Business Care?* Missoula, USA: Conscious Pursuits Inc.

Wigglesworth, C. 2004. 'An Integral Approach to Global Awakening'. *Kosmos* 3(2):30–44.

Wigglesworth, C. 2012. *The Twenty One Skills of Spiritual Intelligence.* New York: Selectbooks, Inc.

Wink, P., and Dillon, M. 2002. 'Spiritual Development across the Adult Life Course: Findings from a Longitudinal Study'. *Journal of Adult Development* 9:79–94.

Wolman, R. 2001. *Thinking with Your Soul: Spiritual Intelligence and Why It Matters.* New York: Harmony.

Wong, P. 1989. 'Successful Aging and Personal Meaning'. *Canadian Psychology* 30:516–525.

Worthington, E., and Sandage, S. 2001. 'Religion and Spirituality'. *Psychotherapy* 38:473–478.

Zika, S., and Chamberlain, K. 1992. 'On the Relation between Meaning in Life and Psychological Well-Being'. *British Journal of Psychology* 83:133–145.

Zohar, D. 1997. *Rewiring the Corporate Brain: Using the New Science to Rethink How We Structure and Lead Organizations.* San Francisco, USA: Berret-Koehler Publishers.

Zohar, D. 2001. *SQ-Spiritual Intelligence: The Ultimate Intelligence.* New York: Bloomsbury.

Zohar, D., and Marshall, I. 2001. *SQ: Connecting with Our Spiritual Intelligence.* New York: Bloomsbury.

Part III

Motherhood and spirituality

6   Research on the lived spirituality of motherhood

Over the past six decades, there has been a growing body of scientific research suggesting connections between religion, spirituality and both mental and physical health. There have also been numerous studies on postpartum anxiety/stress and maternal anxiety during the transition to motherhood. In addition, there has been a particular focus on the effects of psychological disorders amongst women in the postnatal period. Many studies have investigated the neurological causes and biological changes at this point. Most of this research is embedded in the current biomedical model of health.

There is, however, a lack of research on the spirituality of the birthing woman and the academic literature seems to be at the embryonic stage in relation to spirituality and motherhood. A literature survey on the parameters of motherhood and spirituality will help to indicate the progress that spirituality has made in maternal research literature over the last 30 years.

Current research on lived spirituality of motherhood

The survey (Table 6.1) extends from the end of the 1980s to the present day. It summarises each article study (1988–2015) by author, title, participants, themes/findings and theory base. The theory base in the table highlights the different frameworks in which the article is embedded: transpersonal, anthropological, philosophical, health/midwifery, phenomenology, feminism, holism, religion, etc.

It is important to note that there are only a few studies at the early period (Baker 1992; Balin 1988; Callister *et al.* 1999; Corrine *et al.* 1992; Sered 1991) and that academic interest did not seem to seriously emerge until the beginning of the twenty-first century. In 1988, the first ethnographic study was undertaken, focusing on the sacred dimensions of pregnancy and birth. It was conducted from an anthropological and sociological point of view (Balin 1988). Other early studies started giving attention to the cultural and spiritual meanings of the childbirth experience. Birth was analysed as a sacred status and a rite of passage (Baker 1992; Sered 1991). There was also an increased understanding of the significant role of the midwife as the helper in the transition to motherhood and the birth process. In the 1990s, studies began to concentrate on midwifery and

Table 6.1 A literature survey of spirituality in the context of motherhood

Study #	Author/year	Title	Participants	Themes/findings[1]	Theory base
1	Balin (1988)	The Sacred Dimensions of Pregnancy and Birth	Interviewed four women (six/seven months pregnant) and two women who had recently given birth.	*Themes*: exploratory study on ways pregnant women in America are of sacred status and rite of passage. *Findings*: • Changes in physical and social status. • Women's birth rituals. • Changes in their dietary and hygienic habits (sacralising behaviours, attitudes and beliefs).	• Anthropology • Sociology • Transpersonal orientation (ritual/beliefs)
2	Sered (1991)	Childbirth as a Religious Experience? Voices From an Israeli Hospital	Interview of 55 Jewish postpartum women in a maternity hospital in Jerusalem.	*Themes*: exploratory study on the types of religious imagery, language and rituals used by some women in speaking about birth. *Findings*: • 49/55 women performed fertility/childbirth rituals. • Women felt empowered by childbirth. (Jewish law views childbirth as polluting.)	• Religious studies • Anthropology • Feminism • Transpersonal orientation (ritual/beliefs)
3	Corrine *et al.* (1992)	The Unheard Voices of Women: Spiritual Interventions in Maternal-Child Health	Essay article.	*Theme*: discussion on how midwives can learn to assess mothers' spiritual dimensions to overcome crisis in pregnancy or birth. Reviewed different assessments that nurses can use in helping the new mother to cope with her new status and overcoming any crisis (stillbirth, miscarriage, etc.).	• Midwifery • Spirituality and health • Spiritual crisis and disruption

4	Baker (1992)	The Shamanic Dimensions of Childbirth	Fieldwork among the Navajo Indians in North America.	*Themes:* exploratory study on the Shamanic tradition and its advantages for pregnancy and childbirth of the Navajo Indians. *Findings:* • Found aspects that psychotherapists and midwives can learn from these rituals, such as: body integrity, creative visualisation (essential to shamanic healing). • Benefits on how the shamanic midwife offers a perinatal ritual to address the unconscious and guide the pregnant woman through her greatest fears.	• Anthropology • Shamanism • Transpersonal orientation (healing rituals, archetypal, symbolic) • Spiritual intelligence capacities: creativity, conscious awareness and embodiment
5	Callister *et al.* (1999)	Cultural and Spiritual Meanings of Childbirth: Orthodox Jewish and Mormon Women	Interviews with 30 Canadian Orthodox Jewish and 30 American Mormon women.	*Themes:* descriptive, phenomenological study investigated the cultural and spiritual meanings of the childbirth experience from personal perspectives. *Findings:* • Participants expressed codified belief systems of the primary importance of bearing children in obedience to religious law. • The importance of personal connectedness with others and God and the spiritual and emotional dimensions of their childbirth experiences.	• Phenomenology • Holistic nursing • Spiritual intelligence capacity: spiritual meaning production
6	Ayers-Gould (2000)	Spirituality in Birth: Creating Sacred Space Within the Medical Model	Essay.	*Themes:* discussion on the holistic model of pregnancy and birth. Outlined the integration of the cognitive (psychology, intelligence), the physical (the body) and the spirit (beliefs, sacred/symbolic). Also argued the transcendence dimension of birth as a container of hope. Finally, encouraged maternal education devoted to the emotional and spiritual aspects of birth as part of the standard prepared childbirth programmes.	• Holistic nursing • Transpersonal/ transcendence aspects • Spirituality and health • Midwifery

continued

Table 6.1 Continued

Study #	Author/year	Title	Participants	Themes/findings[1]	Theory base
7	Budin (2001)	Birth and Death: Opportunities for Self-Transcendence	Essay paper.	*Themes*: discussion on the nature of self-transcendence in natural birth. Philosophical discussion on birth as normal, natural and healthy (birth as a complete surrender of the woman's body and will, dissolving her ego, ideas and familiar sense of self). Outlined the importance of no fear of dying because there was no 'self' left to resist and fear (transcendent moment of the spiritual birth of woman into mother).	• Transpersonal orientation (self-transcendence) • Natural birth • Philosophy/ psychology/spirituality of birth
8	Bartlett (2001)	Building Sacred Traditions in Birth	Essay paper.	*Themes*: discussion on building a birthing community through traditional and holistic midwifery. Outlined the importance of viewing birth as a sacred event able to raise the state of consciousness through this experience.	• Traditional/holistic midwifery • Spiritual capacities: conscious awareness
9	Hall (2002)	Spiritual Care for Childbirth – Is this the Weakest Link?	Essay article.	*Themes*: analysed the role of midwife and mother to encourage discussion to improve links between all professions involved in the care of women and their babies. Related holism and nursing and the relationship between spiritual elements and care.	• Holistic midwifery • Spirituality and health • Spiritual care in childbirth

No.	Title	Type	Themes/Findings	Key themes
10	The Sacred Place of Birth	Essay.	*Themes*: study analyses the views and values women have of pregnancy and birth and the powerful, spiritual relationship they have with the unborn. *Findings*: • Women's value on the sanctity of pregnancy and birth. • Spiritual nature of the unborn should be recognised.	• Philosophy of birth • Holistic nursing • Spiritual capacity of making meaning production of birth
	Hall (2003)			
11	Motherhood and Spirituality: Faith Reflections From the Inside	Briefing article.	*Themes*: discussion on how to situate motherhood in relation to spirituality in its historical context and to explore ways of bringing the two together. Related the difference between second- and third-wave feminism understanding of motherhood. Outlined how motherhood is integral to the identity of women.	• Eco-feminism • Psychospiritual understanding of motherhood • History/spirituality
	Holness (2004)			
12	The Effects of Islam and Traditional Practices on Women's Health and Reproduction	Questionnaire of 138 household members residing in the territory of three primary healthcare centre in Turkey.	*Themes*: investigated the effects of Islam as a religion and culture on Turkish women's health. *Findings*: • Women's health behaviour changed from traditional to rational as education levels increased. • Religious, traditional attitudes and behaviours predominant in countryside, especially associated with pregnancy/delivery.	• Religion/spirituality and health • Women's health • Islamic tradition
	Bahar *et al.* (2005)			
13	Ancient Mother Goddesses and Fertility Cults in Mothering, Religion and Spirituality	Essay paper.	*Themes*: examined the origins of the concept 'mother goddess', analysed the visual and written material about ancient Eastern Mediterranean goddesses and how they have represented motherhood and fertility in the form of a universal Great Mother or Mother Earth.	• Anthropology/archaeology • History/philosophy of motherhood spiritual representation
	Stuckey (2005)			

continued

Table 6.1 Continued

Study #	Author/year	Title	Participants	Themes/findings[1]	Theory base
14	Klassen (2005)	The Infertile Goddess: A Challenge to Maternal Imagery in Feminist Witchcraft in Mothering, Religion and Spirituality	Personal account as a feminist witch dealing with infertility.	*Themes:* analysed the image of Mother Goddess and the romanticisation of mothering found in feminist witchcraft. Argued that while the Mother Goddess is limited to one type of female experience, and feminist witchcraft is relevant to a large range of women and their varied experiences, multiple Goddess images must be developed and utilised, including the infertile Goddess.	• Feminism and spirituality • Wiccan spirituality • Transpersonal orientation (archetypes, maternal symbols)
15	Villanueva (2005)	Mother Love in Buddhism	Essay.	*Theme:* examined and analysed the love of mother idealised in Buddhist suttas and writings of the bodhisattva parth. Analysed the power of transformation and awakening in motherhood in relation to patriarchal constructs. Outlined the role of compassion, acceptance and love in motherhood and Buddhist philosophy.	• Buddhist philosophy • Feminism/Buddhism (spiritual capacities)
16	Fisher and Bickel (2005)	Awakening the Divine Feminine: A Stepmother-Daughter Collaborative Journey Through Art-Making and Ritual in Mothering, Religion and Spirituality	Dialogue between two women.	*Theme:* dialogical journey with the divine feminine through art, ritual, poetry and reflective writing. Recounted the transpersonal understanding and spiritual awakening for the connection of these two women.	• Feminism account • Autoethnographic • Transpersonal orientation (art/ritual inquiry) • Spiritual emergence (awakening)

	Author (year)	Type	Themes	
17	Sempruch (2005)	The Sacred Mothers, the Evil Witches and the Politics of Household in Toni Morrison's Paradise in Mothering, Religion and Spirituality	Essay.	*Themes*: analysed the negotiation between the sacred and the heretic spaces of culture (theories of Julia Kristeva/Catherine Clement) of women from sociopolitical structures of power, phallocentric authority with spiritual values of the maternal (figure of Consolata).	• Spirituality/psychoanalysis/feminism • Cultural/social studies • Transpersonal orientation (maternal symbols, symbols, archetypes)
18	VanderBerg (2005)	Witnessing Dignity: Irigaray on Mothers and the Divine in Mothering, Religion and Spirituality	Essay.	*Themes*: analysed the recognition of full humanity of our mothers and open up the spiritual realm to women by the interweave between Irigaray's writings and feminine genealogies.	• Feminism/psychoanalysis • Philosophy • Maternal ambivalence and spirituality
19	Duncan (2005)	Hard Labour: Religion, Sexuality and the Pregnant Body in Mothering, Religion and Spirituality	Essay.	*Themes*: analysed the contradictory positioning of black women in pregnancy and economic, political and psychic crises. Discussed images of African pregnant bodies as overly fecund, wild and animalistic.	• Cultural/African narratives • Spirituality/disruption/crisis
20	Hall (2006)	Spirituality at the Beginning of Life	Literature review.	*Themes*: a review of the historical, philosophical and religious views of the spirit of the foetus. Investigation was made of views of the timing of 'ensoulment'. Demonstrated the value women place on the sacredness of pregnancy and birth.	• Holistic nursing • Spirituality and philosophy of the unborn • Spirituality and health

continued

Table 6.1 Continued

Study #	Author/year	Title	Participants	Themes/findings[1]	Theory base
21	Price et al. (2006)	Spirituality and High-Risk Pregnancy: Another Aspect of Patient Care	Interviewed 12 women admitted for high-risk pregnancy complications.	*Themes*: study uncovered the spiritual beliefs and practices of women experiencing high-risk pregnancies. *Findings*: highlighted that within the challenges of a high-risk pregnancy, women often struggled to define their spirituality but recognised spiritual expression as key to healing. Women identified aspects of spirituality that enabled them and to deal with stress of their high-risk pregnancy experience, which they believed enhanced outcomes for themselves and their unborn child.	• Spirituality/crisis/ disruption • Spirituality/health • Spiritual capacity: making meaning/ different knowledge/ language
22	Jesse et al. (2007)	The Effect of Faith or Spirituality in Pregnancy	Interviewed 130 urban low-income pregnant women.	*Themes*: how faith/spirituality affect pregnancy in these particular women. *Findings*: • 47% women in this study described how spirituality affected their pregnancy positively for guidance and support, protection, blessing, or reward, communication with God, strength and confidence, help with difficult moral choices and a generalised positive effect. • 45% described that spirituality did not affect them. • 5.4% were unsure.	• Holistic nursing • Spirituality and health • Spiritual capacity: making meaning production in relation to pregnancy

23	Moloney (2007)	Dancing with the Wind: A Methodological Approach to Researching Women's Spirituality Around Menstruation and Birth	Focus groups, in-depth interviews and autoethnography.	*Themes:* analysed the dimensions of female spirituality connected with the processes of menstruation and birth. *Findings:* • Women as integral human beings (comfortable with their bodies and extraordinary spiritual potential). • Inseparability of body/voice and mind/thought.	• Feminism • Autoethnography • Spiritual capacity of conscious awareness (embodied knowing)
24	Lahood (2007)	Rumour of Angels and Heavenly Midwives: Anthropology of Transpersonal Events and Childbirth	A collection of stories from mothers, fathers and midwives who had participated in transpersonal events during childbirth (from 2001–2006).	*Themes:* compared the local women's non-ordinary state of consciousness (NOSC) with ethnographic accounts of spirit-possession, its relationship to indigenous midwifery and reconstruction the witch-hunts of Medieval Europe from this perspective. *Findings:* • Found the need to revalorise NOSC among birth-giving mothers, and to educate birth attendants in this field. • Midwives are encouraged to learn to identify and support women's NOSC during labour and birth as many women find strength and wisdom by passing through these states in labour.	• Anthropology • Transpersonal psychology • Spiritual capacity (consciousness awareness) • Traditional midwifery
25	Mann et al. (2007)	Religiosity, Spirituality, and Depressive Symptoms in Pregnant Women	Depression was measured using the Edinburgh Postnatal Depression Scale (EPDS) in pregnant women in three obstetrics practices.	*Themes:* cross-sectional study evaluating religiosity, spirituality and depressive symptoms. *Findings:* • 28 women (8.1%) scored above the recommended EPDS cut-off score. Religiosity/spirituality was significantly associated with fewer depressive symptoms.	• Spirituality and health • Crisis/spirituality and disruption

continued

Table 6.1 Continued

Study #	Author/year	Title	Participants	Themes/findings[1]	Theory base
26	Mann et al. (2008)	Do Antenatal Religious and Spiritual Factors Impact the Risk of Postpartum Depressive Symptoms?	Cohort study of women receiving prenatal care obstetrics practices. A six-week follow up postpartum clinic visit. Four measures of religiosity and two measures of spirituality were assessed at baseline.	*Themes*: investigated the association between antenatal religiosity/spirituality and postpartum depression, controlling for antenatal depressive symptoms, social support and other potential confounders. *Findings:* • 36 women (11.7%) scored above the EPDS screening cut-off. • Women who participated in organised religious activities at least a few times a month were markedly less likely to exhibit high depressive symptom scores. • Religious participation assists in coping with the stress of early motherhood.	• Spirituality and health • Crisis/spirituality and disruption
27	Parrat (2008)	Territories of the Self and Spiritual Practices During Childbirth	Book chapter.	*Themes:* • Ordinary practices of life that encircle childbirth as a peak spiritual experience (spiritual practices). • Outlines background concepts to the theory. • Offers a portion of the theory called 'Territories of the Self'.	• Spirituality/nursing • Embodied consciousness (spiritual capacity)
28	Page et al. (2009)	Does Religiosity Affect Health Risk Behaviors in Pregnant and Postpartum Women?	Data from the National Survey of Family Growth.	*Themes*: examined the association between religious involvement and health risk behaviours such as smoking, drinking, marijuana use. *Findings:* • Religious attendance emerged as an important correlate of less risky health behaviours among this nationwide sample of pregnant and postpartum women.	• Spiritual/religion and health • Crisis/disruption/ spirituality

				Themes and Findings	
29	Callister (2010)	Spirituality in Childbearing Women	Literature review.	*Themes*: analysed existing narrative data from cross-cultural studies of childbearing women. *Findings*: • Use of religious beliefs and rituals as powerful coping mechanisms. • Childbirth as a time to make religiosity more meaningful. • The significance of a higher power in influencing birth outcomes. • Childbirth as a spiritually transforming experience.	• Spirituality and health • Cultural narratives ‣ Transpersonal orientation (rituals) • Spiritual ability: transformation
30	Akerjordet (2010)	Being in Charge – New Mothers' Perceptions of Reflective Leadership and Motherhood	Interview with ten new mothers on day 2–3 after giving birth.	*Themes*: analyse new mothers' perceptions of reflective leadership in relation to motherhood. *Findings*: • Being a good mother by reflecting and developing self-identity. • Managing fear, demands and commitments as a mother. • Having the necessary resources to act and lead as a mother. • Believing and trusting in others and self as a leader.	• Spiritual capacity: self-reflection • Spirituality and leadership
31	Hunter *et al.* (2011)	Satisfaction and Use of a Spiritually Based Mantram Intervention for Childbirth-Related Fears in Couples	Mixed-methods design, experimental repeated measures with interviews at six-month follow-up was conducted.	*Themes*: study assessed patient satisfaction with the use of a spiritually based (mantram/sacred word) intervention in expectant couples. *Findings*: • Satisfaction was moderate to high (mantram was used for labour pains and uncertainty. Implications included scheduling flexible classes earlier in pregnancy). • Larger randomised study is needed to assess intervention effectiveness.	• Childbirth and spirituality • Spiritual capacity: conscious awareness (meditation/mantram)

continued

Table 6.1 Continued

Study #	Author/year	Title	Participants	Themes/findings[1]	Theory base
32	Snodgrass (2012)	A Psychospiritual Family-Centered Theory of Care of Mothers in the NICU	Lived experience of mother of a VLBW infant.	*Themes*: study examined women's psychological and theological needs drawing on a mother's lived experience. *Findings*: • Developed a psychospiritual, family-centred theory of care to aid chaplains in providing spiritual care to mothers in the neonatal intensive care unit (NICU).	• Psychospiritual orientation • Crisis/spirituality/ disruption • Spirituality/health • Holistic nursing
33	Crowther (2013)	Sacred Space at the Moment of Birth	Hermeneutic phenomenological study that examined the experiences of birth.	*Themes*: study focuses on the experience of sacred space at the moment of birth. *Findings*: • Stories show a powerful and vulnerable space revealed (magical, feelings of connection and transformative). • Birth as an opening of a sacred space.	• Phenomenology • Transpersonal orientation (sacred, symbolic spaces) • Spirituality and personal narratives • Spiritual capacity (transformation/ connection)
34	Hall (2013a)	Developing a Culture of Compassionate Care – The Midwives' Voice	Commentary paper.	*Themes*: discussion of UK new vision launched with the aim to improve midwifery and nursing care (Department of Health 2012). Paper follows on from a consultation on how to address the shortcomings within nursing), though the issues are applicable across all areas of care (compassion, care, competence, etc.).	• Spirituality and nursing • Spiritual capacities (compassionate care)
35	Hall (2013b)	Spiritual Care: Enhancing Meaning in Pregnancy and Birth	Essay.	*Themes*: discussion about spirituality and spiritual care in relation to midwifery practice and birth. Application was made to the education of midwives in the UK including reference to Nursing and Midwifery Council guidance.	• Spirituality and midwifery • Spirituality and health

#	Author (Year)	Title	Method	Themes / Findings	Categories
36	Nuzum *et al.* (2014)	The Provision of Spiritual and Pastoral Care Following Stillbirth in Ireland: A Mixed Methods Study	Semi-structured qualitative interviews with hospital chaplains in Irish maternity units.	*Themes*: this study reviewed how spiritual care is provided to bereaved parents following stillbirth in maternity units in Ireland and the impact of stillbirth on healthcare chaplains. *Findings*: • Provision of spiritual care following stillbirth in Ireland is diverse. • Spiritual care by chaplains who are not professionally trained and accredited potentially impacts quality and depth of care. • Chaplains experience impact and challenge personal faith/belief.	• Spirituality and health • Crisis/spirituality/ disruption • Spiritual/pastoral care
37	Nuzum *et al.* (2015)	The Spiritual and Theological Issues Raised by Stillbirth for Healthcare Chaplains	Chaplains from 85% of maternity units in the Republic of Ireland.	*Themes*: explored spiritual/theological issues raised for healthcare chaplains, ministering to parents following perinatal bereavement. *Findings*: Theological themes raised for chaplains following perinatal death: • Suffering, doubt and presence. • Theological reflection tool in perinatal healthcare ministry.	• Spirituality and health • Crisis/spirituality/ disruption • Spiritual/pastoral care
38	Klobučar (2015)	The Role of Spirituality in Transition to Parenthood: Qualitative Research Using Transformative Learning Theory	Interviews with 12 adult couples making transition to parenthood.	*Themes*: study researches the meaning of transition to parenthood through the lens of transformative learning theory. *Findings*: • Transformative learning occurs in different spheres of life during transition to parenthood. Discussed spiritual dimension of learning, meaning-making production.	• Spirituality and intelligence (meaning-making production and transformative learning)

continued

Table 6.1 Continued

Study #	Author/year	Title	Participants	Themes/findings[1]	Theory base
39	Moloney and Gair (2015)	Empathy and Spiritual Care in Midwifery Practice: Contributing to Women's Enhanced Birth Experiences	Ten interviews and seven focus groups were conducted with 48 women, including mothers, midwives and staff from a women's service.	*Themes:* article highlights women's stories about midwives' empathy and spiritual care or lack thereof during birth. *Findings:* • Midwives' empathy and spiritual care enhanced a solid foundation for confident mothering. • Lack of empathy, compassion or spiritual care were related with more enduring consequences, birth trauma and difficulty bonding with their babies. • Midwives' empathy and spiritual care can play a key role in creating positive birth and mothering experiences.	• Holistic midwifery • Spirituality/ psychology/health • Spiritual capacities (empathy, connection, compassion) • Holistic nursing • Spirituality and personal maternal narratives
40	Crowther and Hall (2015)	Spirituality and Spiritual Care in and Around Childbirth	Discussion paper.	*Themes:* discussion on authors' own studies and other's research focusing on the complex contextual experiences of childbirth related to spirituality in relation to the growing interest in spiritual care assessments and guidelines. *Findings:* • Spiritual care guidelines into midwifery practice do not address the spiritual meaningful significance of childbirth. Spiritual care guidelines do not appear to acknowledge the lived-experience of childbirth as spiritually meaningful. • Spiritual experiences are felt and beckon sensitive and tactful practice beyond words and formulaic questions.	• Spiritual care and childbirth • Spiritual capacity (meaning-making production)

41	Burns (2015)	The Blessingway Ceremony: Ritual, Nostalgic Imagination and Feminist Spirituality	Doctoral fieldwork with 52 home-birthing women across Eastern Australia.	*Themes*: discussion of Blessingway ceremony (alternative baby shower), popular with home-birthing women. It is woman-centred and draws on the power of ritual to evoke a spiritual experience for the pregnant host and her guests.	• Transpersonal orientation (ritual, symbols) • Feminism/spirituality • Birth/spirituality
				Findings:	
				• Spirituality is experienced as a strong connection between women, their relationship with 'nature' and forged via the nostalgic imagination of women through time and space.	
				• Ceremony is significance as a site of potential spiritual empowerment for pregnant and birthing women.	

Note
1 Information is limited in certain articles (themes and findings).

the need for nurses to be educated in the spiritual dimension of childbirth. Corrine *et al.* (1992) discussed how midwives can learn to assess mothers' spiritual dimensions so as to overcome crisis in pregnancy or birth. At the end of the twentieth century, there was a turn towards personal maternal narratives within the academy (Callister *et al.* 1999).

At the start of the new millennium, the theme of birth and spirituality began to move from the biomedical model to a more holistic understanding of health and the birthing woman. A sacred space began to surface within the medical model (Ayers-Gould 2000) and a transpersonal framework in the understanding of spirituality was used to explore the opportunities for the self-transcendence process at work within the mother (Budin 2001).

Since 2001, the theme of birth and spirituality has been increasingly researched within a nursing/midwifery framework (Hall 2001). Jennifer Hall, a midwifery lecturer at Bournemouth University and clinical editor for *The Practising Midwife* journal, has conducted extensive research on the significance of the spiritual dimension in midwifery training (Hall 2002; 2003; 2006; Hall and Mitchell 2007; Hall and Taylor 2004; Hall *et al.* 2009). Most of her articles on spirituality and birth are reviewed in Table 6.1. Her article on developing a culture of compassion (Hall 2013a) illustrates how this quality is a valuable spiritual capacity that can improve midwifery and nursing care. A recent article (Crowther and Hall 2015) advocates for clear spiritual care guidelines to be integrated into midwifery practice, so that midwives are able to address the spiritual significance of childbirth as a meaningful lived-experience. In the survey table, most of the studies listed for 2005 belonged to a volume entitled *Motherhood and Spirituality*, which was published by the *Journal of the Association for Research on Mothering* and produced in conjunction with York University in Ontario, Canada. This is the only association involved in high-quality scholarship on the subject of mothering and motherhood.

Articles in this volume are accounts of motherhood from the Islamic (Bahar *et al.* 2005), Buddhist, Wicca Spirituality and African religions (Fisher and Bickel 2005; Klassen 2005; Sempruch 2005; Stuckey 2005; Villanueva 2005). Most of these studies contain no participants and are primarily literature review essays on the different religious practices and how they affect the maternal transition.

The relationship between spirituality, religion and the maternal body comes into view in some other studies at this time also (Duncan 2005; Moloney 2007). The concept of 'embodied knowing' in the birth, and the transition to motherhood bearing extraordinary spiritual potential, was seen as new territory to be researched. Dr Jenny Parratt, midwife and fellow of the Australian College of Midwives, has done extensive research on the sense of self and embodied knowing of the mother. Her doctoral thesis, 'Feeling like a Genius: Enhancing Women's Changing Embodied Self during First Childbearing', is a profound study of the phenomenological understanding of the pregnant body employing a perceptual and affective lens regarding the holding of knowledge and power in pregnancy. Parratt considers that a person's spirit is expressed through using power that is intrinsic to the embodied self (Parratt 2010). Moloney's (2007) autoethnography research found that women's body/voice and mind/thought were inseparable, and that by being comfortable with their bodies, women opened their bodies' spiritual potential.

In the literature survey, it was also observed that when a 'disruption' or 'crisis' happens to the mother, there may be a spiritual emergence that assists in mediating the difficult experience. Price *et al.* (2006) highlighted that within the challenges of a high-risk pregnancy, women often struggled to define their spirituality, but recognised spiritual expression as key to healing and dealing with stress. Mann *et al.* (2007; 2008) researched the relationship between spirituality, religion and depressive symptoms pre- and postpartum. His findings show that spirituality is significantly associated with fewer depressive symptoms in pregnant women, and that religious participation assisted in coping with the stress of early motherhood. A recent study has researched the development of a psychospiritual, family-centred theory of care to aid chaplains in providing spiritual care to mothers in the Neonatal Intensive Care Unit (NICU). There is a growing literature dealing with pastoral responses at emergency events such as stillbirth, miscarriage and for mothers with HIV and cancer (Kohl 2012; Manning and Radina 2015; Petro 2015; Walulu and Gill 2011). Nuzum *et al.* (2014) have researched the provision of spiritual and pastoral care following stillbirth, and it has been shown that ongoing education and greater support is needed for chaplains.

The transpersonal feature of the birthing event is usually covered in maternal theory literature. An anthropological fieldwork study conducted from 2001 to 2006 collected stories from mothers, fathers and midwives who had participated in transpersonal events of non-ordinary state of consciousness (NOSC) during childbirth (Lahood 2007). Also, Dr Lynn Clark Callister, a nursing professor at Brigham Young University, has spent 20 years researching the cultural and religious perceptions of childbirth. Her latest article, 'Spirituality in Childbearing Women', is a recompilation and analysis of much of the existing narrative data on spirituality in nursing and health science. Her study shows that the use of religious beliefs and rituals are powerful coping mechanisms and that childbirth is frequently a spiritually transforming experience (Callister 2010). Recent studies have also focused on the experience of sacred space at the moment of birth, and the magical feelings of connection and transformation during birth (Crowther 2013). The use of birth rituals/symbols and archetypes are also examined in the literature as powerful tools for potential spiritual empowerment for pregnant and birthing women. Spirituality in other studies was experienced as a strong connection between women and 'nature' (Baker 1992; Balin 1988; Budin 2001; Burns 2015; Klassen 2005; Sered 1991).

Spiritual capacities are also reflected in some studies in the literature review. A study from Norway explored new mothers' perceptions of reflective leadership in relation to motherhood (Akerjordet 2010). Capacities such as self-awareness, reflexivity and introspection help to mediate the new mother's transformation for reflective leadership. Hall (2013a) highlights the significance of developing a culture of compassionate care towards the birthing woman.

Midwives' empathy and compassion can enhance a solid foundation for confident mothering, whereas a lack of empathy, compassion or spiritual care brings about more enduring consequences for women, including birth trauma and difficulty bonding with their babies. Therefore, midwives' empathy and spiritual care can play a key role in creating positive birth and mothering experiences (Moloney and Gair 2015). When taking into account the research done in spirituality and motherhood over nearly three decades, almost half the literature (18 out of 39 studies) identified birth as a spiritual experience. It is described in transpersonal terms, and the impact of birth is clearly elucidated as the beginning of the transition. Many of the remaining themes that emerged concerned the importance and significance of midwives in assisting the birthing woman. Certainly, the role of spirituality and nursing/midwifery is, and continues to be, well researched (Thomson *et al.* 2011). The effectiveness and need for cultivating spiritual capacities by health professionals are emphasised in many studies. In contrast, the spiritual capacities that may help mothers in their transition are less researched and less elucidated in the literature.

Maternal spiritual capacities in literature survey

The literature review provided evidence of some spiritual capacities of spirituality and motherhood. Many of the themes and spiritual capacities emerging in the literature survey of spirituality in the context of motherhood overlap and relate to the five capacities outlined in spiritual intelligence theory, and also with the three themes arising in the pilot study. Thus, it is important to link the three in order to elucidate unique spiritual capacities that can help and assist mothers in their transition.

Spiritual intelligence capacities and the literature survey

The five spiritual capacities emerging from the spiritual intelligence theory were: (1) personal meaning production; (2) consciousness/awareness; (3) self-reflection/reflexivity; (4) creativity; and (5) transpersonal orientation. All of these spiritual capacities are found in the literature survey.

The construction of personal meaning is essential for the mothers to evaluate what they consider appropriate meaningful emotions, desires and beliefs for their emotional adjustment. A very relevant study from Barlow (1997) concluded that in order to preserve the self and the child, the mother generates through reflection a 'self-constructed mothering'. The maternal transition is a 'highly complex emotional process' and it has often been described as a 'psychic crisis' in the lives of women (Buchanan 2003). The importance of emotions to layers of meaning has been researched (Akerjordet 2010). Personal meaning production is the key spiritual capacity for connection with the inner part of being and also to others. Emotional maturity can be suggested as an expression of spiritual intelligence, and its adjustment in negotiating and integrating the experience is paramount for the creation of personal meaning. Personal meaning production is the spiritual capacity that helps to comprehend the insightful interpretation of the experience (Wilber 1997). The literature review highlights the use of the capacity of making meaning production in order to understand different experiences within birth. Callister *et al.* (1999), in their research on Orthodox Jewish and Mormon women, showed how belief systems, cultural and spiritual meanings of the childbirth experience impact on the way in which mothers raise their children, and their personal connectedness with others and God. The meaning that women attach to birth and to the unborn child is extremely relevant if any crisis happens during pregnancy or birth. Hall (2003) has analysed the powerful spiritual relationship that women have with the unborn as a sacred bond. In high-risk pregnancy experiences, women make meaning of the stressful experience by identifying aspects of spirituality that can help them and their unborn child (Price *et al.* 2006). Crowther and Hall (2015) investigated the importance of the meaningful production that mothers attribute to childbirth. The authors of this study advocate for the spiritual meaningful significance of childbirth (lived-experience of mothers) to be acknowledged into spiritual care guidelines.

Conscious awareness is also an important capacity in many studies in the literature survey. Akerjordet (2010) concluded that the transition to motherhood is mediated by increasing self-awareness. Many researchers consider this 'self-awareness' as essential for developing spiritual maturity (Vaughan 1995, Wilber 1996) and this theme also appears in the maternal literature. Mothers also relate to the description of the changes experienced in this transition as 'self-acceptance' and 'expansion of consciousness' (Ayers-Gould 2000). Such expansion is described by Wilber as integration between subjective, objective and inter-subjective modes of consciousness (Wilber 1996). Many studies in the literature viewed birth as a sacred event and outlined the importance of birth in raising a different state of consciousness through the experience (Baker 1992; Bartlett 2001; Hunter *et al.* 2011; Lahood 2007; Moloney 2007). Conscious awareness is interrelated with the inseparability of body/mind/thought and constitutes what has been called 'embodied knowing' through conscious awareness (Parratt 2008). Women described their experiences of becoming a mother in terms of 'power', of 'facing death' and of 'survival'. These experiences are substantially spiritual in nature. Parratt (2010) researched the connection of the body and spirituality. Mothers conceptualise the self as a 'spiritual knowing' in the experience of the 'embodied knowing'. This study connects this 'spiritual knowing' with change and the ability to express the needs of the moment. This concept is about integration and connection and also about an 'intrinsic power' that provides the courage to face the unknown (Parratt 2010). Consciousness embodiment is an important capacity in the transition to motherhood as the body undertakes a major change that can impact it emotionally, physically and spiritually. The body was conceived as a 'biological organism', the 'ground of personal identity' and a 'social construct' (Merleau-Ponty 1962). Spirituality fully involves people's material bodies, not just their minds or spirits (McGuire 2003). Spiritual intelligence implies facing these existential realities in the full embodied experience of giving birth.

Reflexivity and self-reflection are important capacities for the creation of self-meaning within the maternal transition. New mothers' perception of reflective leadership and motherhood is achieved through the essence of self-reflection (Akerjordet 2010). This study also found that transformation and growth within the transition to motherhood is mediated by reflective self-acceptance. The power of reflection helps the new mother to approach, rather than withdraw from the experience (Siegel 2010). Because this spiritual capacity is the one that evokes profound responses of change and adaptation, it is related, in some studies, where the mother undergoes crisis. Price *et al.* (2006) recount the experience of how mothers, through self-reflection on the experience of high-risk pregnancy, are trying to create new knowledge to cope with the stress. Similarly, studies by Mann *et al.* (2007; 2008) show that when mothers are pushed to their limits at the expense of their own needs, depressive symptoms are a reaction to regulate the emotional system. This system is at full capacity during pregnancy and postpartum periods (Akerjordet and Severinsson 2009). The capacity to self-reflect on those emotions is crucial in accepting the entire whole of the experience – both the negative and positive. Inner resources such as intuition and inner knowledge become very relevant in the development of self-kindness, self-forgiveness, self-compassion and self-acceptance. The complexity of the transition to motherhood creates very confusing and conflicting expectations (cultural, historical, economic, family, emotional, etc.) in the life of the new mother. Through self-reflection, mothers make meaning and create conscious priorities in their lives. Thus, women's self-identity in contemporary, Western society is intrinsically related to cultural/historical self-worth. Mothers will negotiate, integrate or withdraw from certain parts of their lives in order to preserve such identity (Emmanuel *et al.* 2008; Halrynjo and Lyng 2009). Undoubtedly, this self-reflection leads to a 'transformation' in the social, cultural, physical and emotional context of the mother (Barlow 1997). This transformation comes from constructive reflection that leads to new solutions, seeing life in different ways and how flexible the mother is in coping with change (Scharmer 2009). Self-reflection will enable the mother to shift from unhealthy to healthy states in a creative manner (Kornfield 2008; Schuldberg 2007).

Creativity is the direct consequence of this capacity and ultimately is the maternal response to a complete change in status in the life of the woman. The powerful experience of creating a new life can awaken a whole restructuration in the mother of how she sees her life and the world. Many forms of creativity can emerge in the transition to motherhood. Many mothers create a 'self-constructed mothering', in which the creation of social networks and meaningful relationships are developed (Hunter *et al.* 2008). Creative capacities are described as: discovering one's personal gifts and strengths, use of imagination or even the bringing of a fresh perspective to situations in one's life (Johnson 2011). Fear is the normal reaction in a challenging situation. Mothers have to deal with much fear from pregnancy, birth and the postpartum periods. The freedom from fears is linked to creativity (Amram 2007). Baker (1992) showed how rituals and creative visualisation benefit the mother in addressing the unconscious and guiding them in their greatest fears. Rituals are creative events that help the mother to find a sense of knowledge and power within herself (Baker 1992; Balin 1988; Burns 2015; Fisher and Bickel 2005; Klassen 2001; Sered 1991). Parratt (2008) developed a theory of 'territories of the self', in which the spiritual practices during childbirth open a creative transformation of the mother's identity that impacts the afterbirth and daily activity of living. Creative potential is a latent form of power that over time will or will not be actualised. The transition to motherhood is an experiential change. In SQ, creativity is associated with feelings of clarity, connection, opening and energy (Vaughan 2002). Women become aware of experiential change and the disconnection they face with choice after having a baby: maintaining habitual practices or changing the self/ identity. Spirituality practices aim to transcend the ego's rationalisations to dominate. Rational dichotomous thinking disconnects and stops creative energy from emerging (Parratt 2008). The disconnection and disintegrative ways of 'being' can be helped by the use of spiritual practices that foster a sense of connected integration. The metaphor of childbirth has been used by artists for a model of human creativity. This metaphor validates women's artistic effort by unifying their mental and physical labour into pro-creativity (Friedman 1987). A poet expressed this creative power as: 'Thus great with child to speak, and helpless in my throes, Biting my truant pen, beating myself for spite, "Fool", said my muse to me; *look in thy heart, and write*[1] (researcher's emphasis). How the mother will canalise her own creative energy will depend on their responses to the change of 'self/identity' during the transition to motherhood.

The transpersonal orientation is extensively researched in the literature review survey. Many authors analysed pregnancy, childbirth and the transpersonal phenomenon (Ayers-Gould 2000; Baker 1992; Balin 1988; Budin 2001; Burns 2015; Callister 2010; Crowther 2013; Fisher and Bickel 2005; Klassen 2005; Lahood 2007; Sempruch 2005; Sered 1991). Pregnancy, birth and the transition to motherhood have been found to create conditions that are ritualistic in nature and sometimes visionary states have emerged (Davis-Floyd 1992; Klassen 2001; Lahood 2006a; 2006b; Moloney 2006; Tedlock 2005). The psychoanalytic philosopher Kristeva described pregnancy as 'a sort of institutionalised, socialised, natural psychosis' (Kristeva 1997). Mothers have described the birth as 'facing death', 'encountering death' or 'being close to death' (Parratt 2010). Budin (2001) describes birth as a complete surrender of the woman's body and will, dissolving her ego, ideas and familiar sense of self. This study emphasises the importance of no fear of dying because there was no 'self' left to resist and fear. Rituals, archetypes, symbols, art, images are utilised for mothers to make sense of the transition. Carlson comments that:

> In pregnancy and childbirth ... women are gripped by a life-and-death drama that totally destroys an old ego sense of being in control ... they find themselves face-to-face with the Mother as Creator and Destroyer (archetypically) manifesting in irrational terrors or visions or dreams.
>
> (1990, 89)

The literature survey clearly showed that childbirth is a spiritually transforming experience. The use of rituals is a powerful coping mechanism (Callister 2010) and has the potential for spiritual empowerment for pregnant and birthing women (Burns 2015).

The literature survey demonstrated how these SQ capacities come to the fore in the maternal literature. The same investigation is done with the relationship between the pilot study's themes and literature survey in the next section.

Pilot study themes and literature survey

The pilot study thematic analysis highlighted three themes: crisis, embodiment and transformation. The relationship between maternal crisis and spirituality is investigated in nine studies in the literature review survey (Corrine *et al.* 1992; Duncan 2005; Mann *et al.* 2007; 2008; Nuzum *et al.* 2014; 2015; Page *et al.* 2009; Price *et al.* 2006; Snodgrass 2012). The main crisis in maternity that has been researched in relation to spirituality in the studies included in the literature survey are in pregnancy and birth. Overcoming difficult events such as stillbirth, miscarriage, high-risk pregnancies and experiences in the NICU have been investigated from the perspective of midwives, chaplains and how can they assist these mothers' spirituality, in their maternal crisis. Perinatal spiritual care in times of crisis is under-researched in Ireland and is also diverse. Nuzum *et al.* (2014; 2015) concluded that the provision of maternal spiritual care should be by professionally trained and accredited for healthcare professionals involved in it. Snodgrass (2012) proposed the development of a psychospiritual, family-centred theory of care to help the health professionals in assisting the spiritual needs of the mother's lived experience. A few studies also evaluate maternal crisis and spirituality in terms of antenatal and postpartum depression (Mann *et al.* 2007; 2008). Those studies showed that religiosity/spirituality is significantly associated with fewer depressive symptoms in the mother. The 'crisis' analysed in those studies in the literature survey are very important and prevalent but they could be other maternal 'invisible crises' that can occur antenatally, at the time of birth and postnatality. The pilot study showed how women interviewed developed maternal anxiety, feelings of control, perfectionism and maternal ambivalence as a direct consequence of the transition in itself. Although this 'crisis' does not seem to be as intense as someone experiencing postnatal depression, high-risk pregnancy, stillbirth or miscarriage, these 'crisis' feelings formed part of the subjective maternal experience that most mothers go through at different degrees in the transition. These feelings of maternal crisis and their consequences are under-researched in normal birthing women. As the pilot study showed, intense feelings erupted at a daily basis in the mother: anger, joy, love, shame, guilt, loneliness and sadness. These feelings coexist with the maternal transition and the mother's value system is tested. Spiritual capacities may help in naming these feelings and most importantly may put meaning to these difficult maternal feelings. In the spiritual journey, crisis is described as a quest for wholeness and authentic integrity (Lombardi 2008).

The theme of embodiment in the pilot study is also found in the literature survey. Ayers-Gould (2000), Budin (2001), Moloney (2007) and Parratt (2008) discussed a holistic model of pregnancy and birth. In the pilot study, women voiced the experience of a new connection with their bodies around pain, empowerment, change and sexuality. Budin (2001) discussed pain in natural birth as a complete surrender of the woman's body and will, dissolving the ego and ideas. These studies advocated for a holistic model of pregnancy and birth and the integration of the cognitive, physical and spirit in maternity care. Moloney (2007) viewed as inseparable body/voice and mind/thought. Spirituality is the intersection of body, mind and spirit in human beings (McGuire 2003). All women interviewed in the pilot study spoke of an intense bodily connection and their feelings that this provoked in pregnancy, birth, lactation and the postnatal period. Moloney (2007) found that the integrality of human beings is about being comfortable with the body and the extraordinary spiritual potential that the body has. Parratt's (2008; 2010) studies consider that the mother's spirit emerges through the power of the embodied self.

The phenomenological understanding of the pregnant body employs a perceptual and affective lens regarding the holding of knowledge and power in pregnancy. Parratt considers that a person's spirit is expressed through using power that is intrinsic to the embodied self (Parratt 2010). The embodied self (the inseparable body/mind/thought) constitutes an 'embodied knowing' through conscious awareness (Parratt 2008). This concept is linked with the third theme found in the pilot study: transformation.

The pilot study described the liminal nature of birth and the capacity of spiritual transformation in such space. Metaphorically, the woman enters the underworld of the birth experience and emerges as a new self. Many studies in the literature survey explored the sacred status of the birth rite of passage through spiritual lenses (Baker 1992; Balin 1988; Bartlett 2001; Burns 2015; Callister 2010; Crowther 2013; Hunter *et al.* 2011; Lahood 2007; Sered 1991). In these studies, perinatal and birth rituals are found to be transformative for the new mother. Healing, body integrity, spiritual language and creative visualisation were tools that seemed to guide the mother through conscious and unconscious fears. The mother's state of consciousness is transformed. Lahood 2007 even reported on NOSC. In the pilot study, women recognised the profound experience that they had been through, and how they had been transformed into a new self in the maternal transition. Callister (2010) has investigated childbearing women cross-culturally and found that childbirth is a spiritually transforming experience. This transformation seemed to be mediated by a self-awareness, self-reflection and a self-consciousness in the women interviewed in the pilot study. Akerjordet (2010) found that those capacities of self-awareness and reflexivity helped to mediate the new mother's transformation for reflective leadership.

Thus, the three themes (crisis, embodiment and transformation) are present in many studies in the literature survey of spirituality in the context of motherhood. Crisis seems to appear as a distinctive theme that needs further development in the context of spirituality and maternity.

Spirituality, disruption and emergence in the transition to motherhood

A distinctive theme that kept appearing in the literature, pilot study and spiritual intelligence theory was that of 'crisis' and 'disruption'. Giving birth, and its impact in a life, is enough to create a 'psychic crisis' in some women. The pilot study outlined 'crisis' as an important threshold within the liminal space in the transition. Spiritual intelligence has at its theoretical core the study of spiritual capacities that can help individuals in their existential suffering and crisis in everyday living. The literature review also showed how a crisis can happen within pre-birth and postnatal periods, and the impact that it can have on the mother and her capacity to deal with daily challenges within maternity. Thus, it is beneficial to review the theoretical literature of 'spiritual emergency' and 'spiritual emergence', as related to the transition to motherhood.

Researchers recognise the profound psychological, cultural, social and physical work involved in the transition from womanhood to motherhood. Transition involves both disruption and responses to disruption (Meleis *et al.* 2000). Psychoanalytic work suggests that motherhood's transformative potential can cause a kind of 'psychic crisis' in the lives of women (Buchanan 2003). New profound life events, such as motherhood, will shape the self in its evolution and will also create new 'metaphors of the self' that can help with the integration of the maternal experience (Ruffing 2011). In terms of motherhood, studies to date have shown that this crisis is mostly manifested through an emotional response. Many articles have described conflicting maternal emotions, feelings and physical reactions. At the beginning of pregnancy, expectations seem to be at the root of conflict. The expectations placed upon a new mother can be overwhelming, and women have mixed feelings about this (Liamputtong and Naksook 2003; Manne 2005). Unmet expectations have been implicated in postnatal depression (Beck 2002). Mothers described how 'life was dramatically changed in a way that had not been expected' (Thurtle 2003).

Before a spiritual emergence, the individual goes through a process of spiritual crisis/emergency. Spiritual emergency has been defined as a drastic change in the individual's meaning system (Grof and Grof 1989). 'Spiritual emergency' was a term coined by Stanislav and Christina Grof in the 1960s. The Grofs defined it as:

> A crisis when the process of growth and change becomes chaotic and overwhelming ... their sense of identity is breaking down, that their old values no longer hold true, and their personal realities are radically shifting. In some cases, new realms of mystical and spiritual experience enter their lives. They may feel tremendous anxiety, have difficulty coping with their daily jobs, and relationships, and may even fear for their own sanity.
>
> (1989, 254)

The Grofs described the triggers for spiritual emergency as: loss, trauma, disease, failure, powerful sexual experiences, operations, extreme physical exertion; and for women: childbirth, miscarriage or abortion. Research literature has tended to describe this crisis psychologically as maternal anxiety and post-natal depression. In reality, however, women find themselves in a liminal space when this crisis sets in, and do not wish to pathologise it (Liamputtong 2007). Other studies have described a spiritual crisis/emergency as a form of identity crisis, where an individual experiences drastic changes to his or her meaning system (Turner *et al.* 1985). A spiritual crisis often arises from the inability to create a conceptual framework to understand an experience or the emotional/ physical inability to integrate an experience (Bragdon 1993; 2013). All spiritual development is characterised by conflict and the struggle to reconcile opposing perceptions. Religious and philosophical traditions have singled out inner con-flict as the source and the engine of transition and transformation (Coward 1989). Catherine G. Lucas, founder of UK Spiritual Crisis Network, outlines some key features of spiritual emergency/crisis. These features are: the intensity of experience that can consume the whole being; the difficulty of coping with everyday life; the somatisation of such crisis into physical pains and sensations; the powerful emotions that it evokes; and the sense of falling away, including the sense of self in an ego-death temporarily (Lucas 2011).

In the transition to motherhood, there may often be a difficulty in coping with daily life. Mothers in some studies recounted their daily tasks as surrounded by distortions of time and space: bodily sensations (what they eat, wear or sleep) and cognitive distortions (dichotomous thinking, catastrophising) (Luthar *et al.* 2001; Oberman and Josselson 1996; Weaver and Ussher 1997). An interruption of the self happens in the liminal space in the transition to motherhood. In some maternal studies, this experience is identified as a personal crisis and a type of identity disintegration which threatens the women's sense of self (Callister 2010; Darvill *et al.* 2010). Many maternal studies described the uncertainty, the feel-ings of intense vulnerability and crisis as well as the lack of control experienced by mothers during this process (Barlow 1997; Mann *et al.* 2007; 2008; Nelson 2003). Fear is the most common emotion felt during a spiritual emergency/crisis. It manifests as anxiety, dread or panic. The response to fear makes the mother feel unsafe in her own body or mind. Spiritual development is in essence the transcendence of the ego-self. This can be a terrifying process for the ego-self in human beings over-identified with the ego. At transpersonal levels of conscious-ness, the ego senses will begin to disintegrate, and the common response is 'fear of dying' (at this point psychic/physical death gets blurred). The transpersonal phenomena of the birthing woman have extensively been researched in the maternal literature (Ayers-Gould 2000; Baker 1992; Balin 1988; Budin 2001; Burns 2015; Callister 2010; Crowther 2013; Fisher and Bickel 2005; Klassen 2005; Lahood 2007; Sempruch 2005; Sered 1991). While birth is only the initi-ation of the transition, it is commonly very relevant for how the transition will unfold in the postpartum period.

Lucas (2011) distinguishes three key phases to successfully move through spiritual emergency. The first phase is looking after mind, body and soul. The mother who is going through these experiences needs a caring 'holding' from family, friends and professionals, if necessary. The importance of maternal net-works and support are a key in nurturing the mother through this process. Burnout, anxiety, fear and rigidity are the main enemies in this crisis. Bodies also need restructuring, as sleep and eating patterns are severely impaired in the life of the mother. Creative expression (writing, painting, craftwork, music, etc.) and meditation practices are a channel and ground for all the consuming energies experienced. Lucas (2011) called the second phase the hero's journey. For the mother, her own heroine's journey is the capacity to make sense of the experi-ence without losing the meaning of it. The mother needs to self-reflect on her life prior to the baby, the threshold and the postpartum period. In those three points, her own transition is concentrated uniquely. Approaching with honesty and courage the challenges, the changes, the losses in her own self will open the transformation needed for her journey. Refusal to change, rigidity of thought and the need to 'go back' to the person once she was, hinders this journey and stops the maternal creative potential. In the heroine's journey, many spiritual capa-cities are needed but the qualities of self-forgiveness, self-compassion, self-acceptance and self-reflection are the main mediators.

Out of a crisis/emergency, a spiritual emergence can occur. Describing spir-itual emergence, Steindl-Rast noted that:

> It is a kind of birth to a fuller and deeper life, and in which some areas in your life that were not yet encompassed by this fullness of life are now integrated or challenged to be integrated ... breakthroughs are often very painful, often acute, dramatic and happen on all levels: what we call material, spiritual and bodily.
>
> (1985, 55)

Spiritual emergence is an awakening state and a step to a more expanded way of being: a development of consciousness (Bragdon 1993; 2013; Wilber 1986). Motherhood can be a fertile soil where spiritual emergence may occur. Spiritual emergence is the process of creating a meaningful context to integrate out-of-the-ordinary experiences. This process often involves re-evaluating conceptual frameworks for what is meaningful in life. It usually involves both the body and the emotions (Bragdon 1993; 2013). Themes such as ambivalence, over-identification, regression, repression, hostility and separation, that are implicit in the maternal crisis, are intrinsic to spiritual emergence. The mother needs to find ways to maintain physical, emotional and spiritual stability in the face of the crisis. In spiritual emergence, archetypes and symbols are quite relevant in vali-dating the profound psychological renewal. Psychospiritual emergence can result in emotional and psychosomatic healing, remarkable psychological transforma-tion and consciousness evolution (Grof 1998; Grof and Grof 1989). The psyche will transform and expand into a different conceptual framework. These experi-ences are often described as leading to 'an expanded consciousness'. Archetypes often seem to impact on the psyche. Carl Jung is the father of investigations of how archetypes help in the understanding of the psyche (Jung 1967). On becoming a mother, a powerful, central archetype is awakened in women: the creator and the destroyer. The conflict between both archetypes emerges into maternal ambivalence. The way this ambivalence is negotiated will depend on the extent of the inner depth to which the mother is willing to go. The use of rituals for the mother, as shown in the maternal literature, acts as intermediary between spiritual emergence and transformation (Klassen 2001; Lahood 2006a; 2006b; Moloney 2006; Tedlock 2005).

Spiritual emergence also happens at a bodily level. As explained earlier, with 'embodied consciousness', the mother undergoes a whole physical change. Embodiment is related to the spiritual, psychological and physiological elements of the mother. It is described as the bodily expression of spirit, as the corporeal habitation of the soul and as a unifying force (Trumble and Stevenson 2002). The body has been understood as being disconnected from the mind, spirit and social and cultural context in medicine and modernity. It is an isolated object (Davis-Floyd 1992). These cultural ideas will impact on the mother's sense of her body. The maternal body undergoes a crisis as the boundaries between the self and the other are already troubled. The woman's body nurtures another human being within. The boundaries between self and environment also become altered and the body needs to respond to its environment according to the psychological, cultural and spiritual make-up of the mother (Davis and Walker 2008).

The feminine body has already entered this process in a state of conflict. Descartes elaborated a theory of personhood that was characterised by a mind/body split that has come to be known as 'Cartesian dualism' (Bowie *et al.* 2007). Up to this time, there is a polarisation of mind and body in Western philosophy (McCann and Kim 2003). Also, at birth, the mother's body competes between two different discourses: the biomedical versus the natural birth. Both discourses can deepen into extremes and have the potential to become oppressive tyrants, discourses for the future mother (Coslett 1994; Murphy-Lawless 1998). These conceptualisations will create a conflict in the woman's body and can cause a sense of failure when the woman's 'womanhood' and 'motherhood' are called into question. The study of the spiritual dimension in the birthing woman must accept the uniqueness of each woman's embodied experience. Women often feel decontextualised from their lived, embodied experiences, and this decontextualisation has the potential to destroy their freedom and their capacity for self-change (Grosz 1994; 1995). This decontextualisation can fuel the embodied crisis in the transition to motherhood.

The maternal literature revealed how the pain of childbirth has been considered to be connected with the power and control of the woman's body. The opening of the cervix has been related to the opening of the self (Hall *et al.* 2009). Many women have expressed how giving birth for the first time was, in many ways, a rebirth (Callister *et al.* 2001). Some women described their 'connected' body experience with the power of creation (Johnson *et al.* 2007).

Empowerment is at the core of the woman's embodied self as who she is or what she can become (Parratt 2008).

The end of the heroine's journey is the reward. The reward may be an experience of profound grace, deep insight into the nature of reality or a new-found self. The end of the journey is always a new beginning, a rebirth. This is the opening in which transformation happens. Many mothers find a whole restructuring of priorities, family, friends and work. The way they want to express themselves in the world can changes to something new. The inner transformation manifests into an outer transformation with inner drive to achieve goals, personal growth and development towards self-actualisation (Siegel 2010).

King's seminal study on women and spirituality affirmed that: 'motherhood is a rich and widely ramified concept linked to biological birth, to culturally learned patterns of mothering and to expression of ... spiritual insights of human experience' (King 1989, 79).

After the initial pilot study and maternal literature review, a further set of interviews were conducted with seven mothers. Experience is a subjective appreciation of what it is going on internally during a particular moment in time. But experience also has a longer-term meaning of inner events in which the internal experience, with time, is transformed into a way of daily living for the person. It is paramount to hear the 'voices' of these mothers in their own maternal transition. In the next chapter, seven narratives are weaved from the interviews into unique stories in the transition to motherhood.

Note

1 Extract from the poem 'Astrophil and Stella I' by Sir Philip Sidney 1591 (Cooper 1968).

References

Akerjordet, K. 2010. 'Being in Charge – New Mothers' Perceptions of Reflective Leadership and Motherhood'. *Journal of Nursing Management* 18(4):409–417.

Akerjordet, K., and Severinsson, E. 2009. 'Emotional Intelligence, Reactions and Thoughts: Part 2: A Pilot Study'. *Nursing Health Science* 11(3):213–220.

Amram, Y. 2007. *The Seven Dimensions of Spiritual Intelligence: An Ecumenical Grounded Theory*. Paper presented at the 115th annual conference of the American Psychological Association, San Francisco, USA, August 2007.

Ayers-Gould, J. 2000. 'Spirituality in Birth: Creating Sacred Space within the Medical Model'. *International Journal of Childbirth Education* 15(1):14–17.

Bahar Z., Okcay, S., Ozbicakci, A., Beser, B., and Ozturk, M. 2005. 'The Effects of Islam and Traditional Practices on Women's Health and Reproduction'. *Nursing Ethics* 12(6):557–570.

Baker, J. 1992. 'The Shamanic Dimensions of Childbirth'. *Pre- and Peri-natal Psychology Journal* 7(1):5–20.

Balin, J. 1988. 'The Sacred Dimensions of Pregnancy and Birth'. *Qualitative Sociology* 11(4):275–301.

Barlow, C. 1997. 'Mothering as a Psychological Experience: A Grounded Theory Exploration'. *Canadian Journal of Counselling* 31(3):232–237.

Bartlett, W. 2001. 'Building Sacred Traditions in Birth'. *Midwifery Today* 58: 24–26.

Beck, C. 2002. 'Postpartum Depression: A Metasynthesis'. *Qualitative Health Research* 12(4):453–472.

Bowie, B., Michaels, M., and Solomon, R. 2007. *Twenty Questions. An Introduction to Philosophy.* Fort Worth, USA: Harcourt Brace.

Bragdon, E. 1993. *Helping People with Spiritual Problems.* Vermont, USA: Lightening Up Press.

Bragdon, E. 2013. *The Call of Spiritual Emergency.* San Francisco, USA: Harper and Row Publishers.

Buchanan, A. J. 2003. *Mother Shock: Tales from the First Year and Beyond – Loving Every (Other) Minute of It.* Emeryville, USA: Seal Press.

Budin, W. 2001. 'Birth and Death: Opportunities for Self-Transcendence'. *Journal Perinatal Education* 10(2):38–42.

Burns, E. 2015. 'The Blessingway Ceremony: Ritual, Nostalgic Imagination and Feminist Spirituality'. *Journal of Religious Health* 54(2):783–797.

Callister, L. 2010. 'Spirituality in Childbearing Women'. *Journal of Perinatal Education* 19(2):16–24.

Callister, L., Semenic, S., and Foster, J. 1999. 'Cultural and Spiritual Meanings of Childbirth: Orthodox Jewish and Mormon Women'. *Journal of Holistic Nursing* 17(3):280–295.

Callister, L., Vehvilainen-Julkunen, K., and Lauri, S. 2001. 'Giving Birth: Perceptions of Finnish Childbearing Women'. *The American Journal of Maternal Child Nursing* 36:28–32.

Carlson, K. 1990. *In Her Image: The Unhealed Daughter's Search for Her Mother.* Colorado, USA: Shambhala.

Cooper, Sherod M. 1968. *The Sonnets of Astrophil and Stella: A Stylistic Study.* The Hague, The Netherlands: Mouton.

Corrine, L., Bailey, V., Valentin, M., Morantus, E., and Shirley, L. 1992. 'The Unheard Voices of Women: Spiritual Interventions in Maternal-Child Health'. *The American Journal of Maternal Child Nursing* 17(3):141–145.

Coslett, T. 1994. *Women Writing Childbirth. Modern Discourses of Motherhood.* Manchester, UK: Manchester University Press.

Coward, R. 1989. *The Whole Truth: The Myth of Alternative Health.* London: Faber & Faber.

Crowther, S. 2013. 'Sacred Space at the Moment of Birth'. *Practical Midwife* 16(11):21–23.

Crowther, S., and Hall, J. 2015. 'Spirituality and Spiritual Care in and around Childbirth'. *Women and Birth* 28(2):173–178.

Darvill, R., Skirton, H., and Farrand, P. 2010. 'Psychological Factors that Impact on Women's Experiences of First-Time Mothers: A Qualitative Study of the Transition'. *Midwifery* 26:357–366.

Davis, D., and Walker, K. 2008. 'Re-discovering the Maternal Body in Midwifery through an Exploration of Theories of Embodiment'. *Midwifery* 32(3):486–501.

Davis-Floyd, R. 1992. *Birth as an American Rite of Passage.* Oakland, USA: University of California Press.

Department of Health. 2012. *Compassion in Practice.* www.england.nhs.uk/wp-content/uploads/2012/12/compassion-in-practice.pdf.

Duncan, C. 2005. 'Hard Labour: Religion, Sexuality and the Pregnant Body in Mothering, Religion and Spirituality'. *Journal of the Association for Research on Mothering* 7(1):167–173.

Emmanuel, E., Creedy, D., St. John, W., Gamble, J., and Brown, C. 2008. 'Maternal Role Development following Childbirth among Australian Women'. *Journal of Advanced Nursing* 64:18–26.

Fisher, V., and Bickel, B. 2005. 'Awakening the Divine Feminine: A Stepmother-Daughter Collaborative Journey through Art-Making and Ritual in Mothering, Religion and Spirituality'. *Journal of the Association for Research on Mothering* 7(1):52–67.

Friedman, S. 1987. 'Creativity and the Childbirth Metaphor: Gender Difference in Literary Discourse'. *Feminist Studies* 13(1):49–82.

Grof, S. 1998. 'Ken Wilber's Spectrum Psychology: Observations from Clinical Consciousness Research'. In *Ken Wilber in Dialogue: Conversations with Leading Transpersonal Thinkers*, edited by D. Rothberg and S. Kelly, 85–115. Wheaton, USA: Quest Books.

Grof, S., and Grof, C. 1989. *Spiritual Emergency: When Personal Transformation Becomes a Crisis.* New York: TarcherPerigee.

Grosz, E. 1994. *Volatile Bodies. Toward a Corporeal Feminism.* Bloomington, USA: Indiana University Press.

Grosz, E. 1995. *Space, Time and Perversion. Essays on the Politics of Bodies.* New York: Routledge.

Hall, J. 2001. *Midwifery Mind and Spirit: Emerging Issues of Care.* Oxford, UK: Books for Midwives.

Hall, J. 2002. 'Spiritual Care for Childbirth – Is This the Weakest Link?'. *Spirituality and Health* 3:37–40.

Hall, J. 2003. 'The Sacred Place of Birth'. *Midwifery Today* 66:11–22.

Hall, J. 2006. 'Spirituality at the Beginning of Life'. *Journal of Clinical Nursing* 15(7):804–810.

Hall, J. 2013a. 'Developing a Culture of Compassionate Care – The Midwives' Voice?'. *Midwifery* 29(4):269–271.

Hall, J. 2013b. 'Spiritual Care: Enhancing Meaning in Pregnancy and Birth'. *Practical Midwife* 16(11):26–27.

Hall, J., and Taylor, M. 2004. 'Birth and Spirituality'. In *Normal Childbirth: Evidence and Debate*, edited by S. Downes, 41–56. Edinburgh, UK: Churchill Livingston.

Hall, J., and Mitchell, M. 2007. 'Teaching Spirituality to Student Midwives: A Creative Approach'. *Nurse Education in Practice* 7(6):416–424.

Hall, W., Hauck, Y., Carty, E., Hutton, E., Fenwick, J., and Stoll, K. 2009. 'Childbirth Fear, Anxiety, Fatigue, and Sleep Deprivation in Pregnant Women'. *Journal of Obstetric, Gynecologic, and Neonatal Nursing* 38(5):567–576.

Halrynjo, S., and Lyng, S. 2009. 'Preferences, Constraints or Schemas of Devotion? Exploring Norwegian Mothers' Withdrawals from High-Commitment Careers'. *The British Journal of Sociology* 60:321–343.

Holness, L. 2004. 'Motherhood and Spirituality: Faith Reflections from the Inside'. *Religion and Spirituality* 18(61):66–71.

Hunter, B., Berg, M., Lundgren, M., Ólafsdóttir, O., and Kirkham, M. 2008. 'Relationships: The Hidden Threads in the Tapestry of Maternity Care'. *Midwifery* 24:132–137.

Hunter, L., Bormann, J., Belding, W., Sobo, E., Axman, J., Reseter, B., and Hanson, Miranda, C. 2011. 'Satisfaction and Use of a Spiritually Based Mantram Intervention for Childbirth-Related Fears in Couples'. *Applied Nursing Research* 24(3):138–146.

Jesse, D., Schoenboom, C., and Blanchard, A. 2007. 'The Effect of Faith or Spirituality in Pregnancy'. *Journal of Holistic Nursing* 25(3):151–158.

Johnson, P. 2011. 'An Atlantic Genealogy of "Spirit Possession"'. *Comparative Studies in Society and History* 53:393–425.

Johnson, T., Callister, L., Freeborn, D., Beckstrand, R., and Huender, K. 2007. 'Dutch Women's Perceptions of Childbirth in the Netherlands'. *The American Journal of Maternal Child Nursing* 32(3):170–177.

Jung, C. 1967. 'Symbols of Transformation (1912)'. In *Collected Works, Volume 5*, translated by R. F. C. Hull. Princeton, USA: Princeton University Press.

King, V. 1989. *Women and Spirituality*. London: Macmillan.

Klassen, P. 2001. *Blessed Events: Religion and the Home Birth Movement in America*. Princeton, USA and Oxford, UK: Princeton University.

Klassen, C. 2005. 'The Infertile Goddess: A Challenge to Maternal Imagery in Feminist Witchcraft in Mothering, Religion and Spirituality'. *Journal of the Association for Research on Mothering* 7(1):45–51.

Klobučar, N. 2015. 'The Role of Spirituality in Transition to Parenthood: Qualitative Research Using Transformative Learning Theory'. *Journal of Religious Health* 15:1–14.

Kohl, K. 2012. 'Remembering Your Faith through the Grief: Experiencing a Miscarriage'. *Journal of Pastoral Care Counselling* 66(1):8.

Kornfield, J. 2008. *The Wise Heart*. New York: Bantam Books.

Kristeva, J. 1997. *The Portable Kristeva*. New York: Columbia University.

Lahood, G. 2006a. 'An Anthropological Perspective on Near-Death-Like Experiences in Three Men's Pregnancy-Related Spiritual Crises'. *Journal of Near-death Studies* 24(4):211–236.

Lahood, G. 2006b. 'Skulls at the Banquet: Near Birth as Nearing Death'. *Journal of Transpersonal Psychology* 38(1):1–24.

Lahood, G. 2007. 'Rumour of Angels and Heavenly Midwives: Anthropology of Transpersonal Events and Childbirth'. *Women and Birth* 20(7):3–10.

Liamputtong, P. 2007. 'When Giving Life Starts to Take the Life out of You: Women's Experiences of Depression after Childbirth'. *Midwifery* 23:77–91.

Liamputtong, P., and Naksook, C. 2003. 'Life as Mothers in a New Land: The Experience of Motherhood among Thai Women in Australia'. *Health Care for Women International* 24:650–668.

Lombardi, N. 2008. 'Dancing in the Underworld: The Quest for Wholeness'. In *She is Everywhere! Vol. 2: An Anthology of Writings in Womanist/Feminist Spirituality*, edited by A. Williams, 337–350. Lincoln, USA: iUniverse.

Lucas, C. 2011. *In Case of Spiritual Emergency: Moving Successfully through Your Awakening*. Forres, UK: Findhorn Press.

Luthar, S., Doyle, K., Suchman, N., and Mayes, L. 2001. 'Developmental Themes in Women's Emotional Experiences of Motherhood'. *Development & Psychopathology* 13(1):165–182.

Mann, J. R., McKeown, R. E., Bacon, J., Vesselinov, R., and Bush, F. 2007. 'Religiosity, Spirituality, and Depressive Symptoms in Pregnant Women'. *International Journal of Psychiatry in Medicine* 37(3):301–313.

Mann, J. R., McKeown, R. E., Bacon, J., Vesselinov, R., and Bush, F. 2008. 'Do Antenatal Religious and Spiritual Factors Impact the Risk of Postpartum Depressive Symptoms?'. *Journal of Women's Health* 17(5):745–755.

Manne, A. 2005. *Motherhood: How Should We Care for Our Children?* Sydney, Australia: Allen and Unwin.

Manning, L., and Radina, M. 2015. 'The Role of Spirituality in the Lives of Mothers of Breast Cancer Survivors'. *Journal of Religion, Spiritual and Aging* 1:27(2–3):125–144.

McCann, C., and Kim, S. eds 2003. *Feminist Theory Reader. Local and Global Perspectives*. New York: Routledge.

McGuire, M. 2003. 'Why Bodies Matter: A Sociological Reflection on Spirituality and Materiality'. *Spiritus: A Journal of Christian Spirituality* 3(1):1–18.

Meleis, A., Sawyer, L., Im, E., Schumacher, K., and Messias, D. 2000. 'Experiencing Transitions: An Emerging Middle Range Theory'. *Advances in Nursing Science* 23(1): 12–28.

Merleau-Ponty, M. 1962. *The Phenomenology of Perception*. New York: Routledge and Kegan Paul.

Moloney, S. 2006. 'The Spirituality of Childbirth'. *Birth Issues* 15:41–46.

Moloney, S. 2007. 'Dancing with the Wind: A Methodological Approach to Researching Women's Spirituality around Menstruation and Birth'. *International Journal of Qualitative Methods* 6(1):114–125.

Moloney, S., and Gair, S. 2015. 'Empathy and Spiritual Care in Midwifery Practice: Contributing to Women's Enhanced Birth Experiences'. *Women Birth* 28(4):323–328.

Murphy-Lawless, J. 1998. *Reading Birth and Death. A History of Obstetric Thinking*. Cork, Ireland: Cork University Press.

Nelson, A. 2003. 'Transition to Motherhood'. *JOGNN* 32:465–477.

Nuzum, D., Meaney, S., and O' Donoghue, K. 2014. 'The Provision of Spiritual and Pastoral Care following Stillbirth in Ireland: A Mixed Methods Study'. *BMJ Supportive Palliative Care*. [Epub ahead of print].

Nuzum, D., Meaney, S., O'Donoghue, K., and Morris, H. 2015. 'The Spiritual and Theological Issues Raised by Stillbirth for Healthcare Chaplains'. *Journal of Pastoral Care and Counselling* 69(3):163–170.

Oberman, Y., and Josselson, R. 1996. 'Matrix of Tensions: A Model of Mothering'. *Psychology of Women Quarterly* 20(3):341–359.

Page, R., Ellison, C., and Lee, J. 2009. 'Does Religiosity Affect Health Risk Behaviors in Pregnant and Postpartum Women?'. *Maternal Child Health Journal*. 13(5):621–632.

Parratt, J. 2008. 'Territories of the Self and Spiritual Practices during Childbirth'. In *Birth Territory and Midwifery Guardianship*, edited by K. Fahy, 39–54. Oxford, UK: Books for Midwives.

Parratt, J. 2010. *Feeling Like a Genius: Enhancing Women's Changing Embodied Self during First Childbearing*. PhD Diss., University of Newcastle, Newcastle, Australia.

Petro, S. 2015. 'Drawing Close to the Brokenhearted: Pastoral Responses to Parents Grieving Stillbirth'. *Journal of Pastoral Care and Counselling* 69(1):13–18.

Price, S., Breen, G., and Lake, M. 2006. 'Spirituality and High-Risk Pregnancy: Another Aspect of Patient Care'. *AWHONN Lifelines* 10(6):466–473.

Ruffing, J. 2011. *To Tell the Sacred Tale*. New York: Paulist Press.

Scharmer, O. 2009. *Theory U Leading from the Future as it Emerges. Open Mind, Open Heart, Open Will. The Social Technology of Presencing*. San Francisco, USA: Berrett Koehler Publishers.

Schuldberg, D. 2007. 'Living Well Creativity: Our Hidden Potential'. In *Everyday Creativity and New Views of Human Nature*, edited by R. Richards, 55–73, Washington, DC: American Psychological Association, 2007.

Sempruch, J. 2005. 'The Sacred Mothers, the Evil Witches and the Politics of Household in Toni Morrison's Paradise in Mothering, Religion and Spirituality'. *Journal of the Association for Research on Mothering* 7(1):98–109.

Sered, S. 1991. 'Childbirth as a Religious Experience? Voices from an Israeli Hospital'. *Journal of Feminist Studies in Religion* 7(2):7–18.

Siegel, D. 2010. *Mindsight, the New Science of Personal Transformation*. New York: Random House.

Snodgrass, J. 2012. 'A Psychospiritual, Family-Centered Theory of Care for Mothers in the NICU'. *Journal Pastoral Care Counsel* 66(1):2.

Steindl-Rast, D. 1985. *In Helping People with Spiritual Problems by E. Bragdon*. Vermont, USA: Lightening Up Press.

Stuckey, J. 2005. 'Ancient Mother Goddesses and Fertility Cults in Mothering, Religion and Spirituality'. *Journal of the Association for Research on Mothering* 7(1):32–44.

Tedlock, B. 2005. *The Woman in the Shaman's Body: Reclaiming the Feminine in Religion and Medicine*. New York: Random House/Bantam.

Thomson, G., Dykes, F., and Downe, S. 2011. *Qualitative Research in Midwifery and Childbirth: Phenomenological Approaches*. London: Routledge.

Thurtle, V. 2003. 'First-Time Mothers' Perceptions of Motherhood and Postnatal Depression'. *Community Practitioner* 76:261–265.

Trumble, W., and Stevenson, A. eds 2002. *The Shorter Oxford English Dictionary, 5th edition*. Oxford, UK: Oxford University Press.

Turner, L., Barnhouse, R., and Lu, F. 1985. 'Religious and Spiritual Problem: A Culturally Sensitive Diagnostic Category in the DSM-IV'. *Journal/Nervous and Mental Disease* 183(7):435–444.

VanderBerg, N. 2005. 'Witnessing Dignity: Irigaray on Mothers and the Divine in Mothering, Religion and Spirituality'. *Journal of the Association for Research on Mothering* 7(1):132–142.

Vaughan, F. 1995. *Shadows of the Sacred: Seeing through Spiritual Illusions*. Wheaton, USA: Quest Books.

Vaughan, F. 2002. 'What is Spiritual Intelligence?'. *Journal of Humanistic Psychology* 42(2):16–33.

Villanueva, K. 2005. 'Mother Love in Buddhism'. *Journal of the Association for Research on Mothering*, 7(1):68–77.

Walulu, R., and Gill, S. 2011. 'Role of Spirituality in HIV-Infected Mothers'. *Issues in Mental Health Nursing* 32(6):382–384.

Weaver, J., and Ussher, J. 1997. 'How Motherhood Changes Life: A Discourse Analytic Study with Mothers of Young Children'. *Journal of Reproductive & Infant Psychology* 15(1):51–68.

Wilber, K. 1986. *Transformations of Consciousness: Conventional and Contemplative Perspectives on Development*. Boston, USA: Shambhala New Science Library.

Wilber, K. 1996. *A Brief History of Everything*. Boston, USA: Shambhala.

Wilber, K. 1997. *The Eye of Spirit: An Integral Vision for a World Gone Slightly Mad*. Boston, USA: Shambhala.

7 Seven narratives of maternal transition

Interviewing had a life of its own. Through questions about their experiences, mothers were invited to tell their maternal stories. Interviews were informal in nature, leaving space for the mothers to explore their own narrative, but at the same time allowing a 'dialogue' with them in a natural manner. There were no set questions to be asked. Every interview was unique as it unfolded, depending on where the mother was going with her narrative.

Mothers lead with their own voices and decided where they wanted to go in terms of telling their own experiences. They talked about all aspects and events surrounding their experiences. This way, each mother 'finds her own voice', which was the real purpose of this kind of human inquiry. It was not about gathering data, but rather, healing the alienation and the split that characterises postmodern experience by actively listening to a unique maternal narrative. Writing someone else's story is an empathetic act. It is daring to 'walk in the mothers' shoes' and use 'intuitive attentiveness' in order to compose individual stories.

At the time of the interview, all mothers were married; three were part-time workers and four were stay-at-home mums. All had third-level educations (university, college or vocational school) and were from middle-class socio-economic backgrounds. Mothers ranged in age from 40 to 57 years, with a median age of 49 years. The median number of children was three, and their median age was 14 years (see Table 7.1).

Table 7.1 Demographic characteristics of research participants

Name (pseudonym)	Age (years)	Number of children	Age of children (years)
Sophia	45	3 (2 boys, 1 girl)	8, 5 and 2
Ann	40	3 (2 girls, 1 boy)	7, 5 and 3
Serena	54	3 (2 boys, 1 girl)	27, 25 and 23
Dana	49	4 (3 boys, 1 girl)	17, 14, 9 and 7
Eve	50	3 (2 boys, 1 girl)	17, 14 and 12
Barbara	57	2 (2 girls)	30 and 27
Clare	46	3 (2 boys, 1 girl)	16, 14 and 12

Seven narratives of maternal transition

Sophia:[1] the difference between what is and what should be is an ocean of anger, frustration and disappointment

Sophia finished her interview with this quotation from an ancient yoga scripture. As a yoga teacher, she has good knowledge of the Yoga Sūtras of Patañjali from Ashtanga Yoga and Hindu philosophy. She included this quotation to represent what she had learned in her transition to motherhood. Her knowledge of yoga will challenge, help and often 'save' her in the process of motherhood. She is in her 40s. She has two boys (aged seven and five years) and a girl (two years). Shortly after she met her partner for the first time, she found that she felt calm and grounded with him. She experienced an intense desire to have a baby with him:

> It was very real, very real and warm and just ... it was just a really, really happy time and I can, you know, remember when I just started to feel like, wanting to have a baby, it was just ... and it wasn't even a sort of thinking, you know, it was like a physical, like my body craving. I feel emotional about it.

The memory of her desire for a new life brought her to tears while she was trying to explain her intense emotions. She took a sharp intake of breath and started talking about the pregnancy and practising and attending yoga courses during that time. Although she had a relatively good first pregnancy, looking back she felt there was a lot going on in her life at the time. She was finishing a three-week residential yoga course and found it emotionally difficult to be away from her partner. Sophia got really sick at this time with *E. coli* from dirty water in the ashram, and that really affected her pregnant body for the rest of the pregnancy. Once home from the course, she had the stress of moving from her partner's mum's house to a different house again. In retrospect, she felt that those last months were not the ideal calm months that she was yearning for. She clearly blamed that disruptive time for the consequent traumatic birth of her first child. A hint of blame could be heard in her words while she was trying to make sense of that time. She concluded that she had felt disconnected from her own body and did not make the time to do antenatal yoga in preparation for the birth. Expectations were very high in her head: '... when I look back on it, I didn't really ... like up here in my head I had read the books and I knew it all and I just thought, "I do yoga, I'll be fine"'.

The birth: intense sense of failure and shock

Sophia, as a yoga teacher, wanted her body to 'respond' to a natural birth experience with little medical intervention. She did not know what to expect, but at the same time had a clear vision of how things should be happening. This theme between how things are and how they should be, is a clear central theme in Sophia's transition to motherhood from prenatal to postnatal experiences.

She was in labour for a long time. The baby was in the occipital position. She experienced very intense pain in her lower back. She was not dilating fast and was in labour for 18 hours. Her birth plans were not to have Pethidine, forceps, ventouse or an epidural. She wanted to have her baby naturally. When exhausted by pain, disappointed by her own body and emotionally destroyed, she felt she could not do it anymore and she asked for an epidural. She described it as follows:

> ... I just got to the point where I was crying, just saying, 'I can't do it anymore, I can't do it,' and had the epidural, and the sense of failure, I just, it was.... I just felt I'd failed myself that I wasn't able to birth my baby the way I wanted to ...

She described the birth experience as traumatic. Through the interview, she mentioned a couple of times how she did not face that trauma until a year later, and that it took her two years to get over it. While she was recalling the whole experience, her own reflections were crucial to the understanding of her narrative.

Sophia felt that the meaning of the traumatic experience made her stronger, more compassionate and a more understanding yoga teacher. Her own failed expectations opened the possibility to challenge perfection within herself that she did not know was that strong. The feelings of sadness and shock that she had to deal with led to a transforming journey. She called it a humbling experience:

> ... there was a sadness, and I suppose there was a kind of shock that it's not just about me deciding how things are ... it wasn't according to my plan at all, and, I suppose, humbling, you know: a humbling experience ...

Transition to motherhood: opening up to a 'new self' and 'new parts of me'

Sophia felt that motherhood was not going according to plan. She related an idyllic image of this wonderful earth mother where she described a scene from a Paula Yates's autobiography:

> ... this scene in the book where, you know, she takes her three beautifully dressed daughters off on a picnic and they just go off on this jaunt and Paula was so beautiful and the daughters were all beautifully dressed, lovely dresses and I remember thinking, 'I want this. It's so me, you know, when I have kids and I ...'. Of course I visualised that I'd have daughters, you know, we'd just go off on adventures and head off in the car, and have such great fun and we'd all be just so happy and I do yoga so my kids will be so calm ...

She was challenged by her first son's personality. He has a sort of oppositional disorder type personality. He argued all the time and had loads of tantrums to the extreme. She felt she could not deal with him and sought counselling for a while. Her own perfection was put to a test: '... I think without even realising it, I guess, I associated control with what you aspire to: being a good parent is being in control...'. Control versus perfection brought the possibility of starting to reflect on the experience in a new way. Sophia thought that letting go of such control and acknowledging that she did not have all the answers, was crucial in the process. She came to the conclusion that motherhood is dealing with constant evolution and change. All the initial doubts on how to parent and how to behave could be transformed through awareness. It was not an easy task, and she had to go through some painful feelings.

During that time, it was clear to her that her identity was being somehow altered. She felt detached from the kind of person she was becoming, to the point of not even recognising herself in a physical way:

> But a few months of kind of saying, 'Yes, I'm fine', and going through the motions, but I wasn't really and I remember one day sort of walking to the shops and pushing R along in the pram, and it was almost as if I had an out-of-body experience: I was looking at this little mammy walking along, pushing the pram, going, 'God, is that me? What am I doing? I don't know what to be doing with myself'. I didn't know what or who I was ...

The acculturation into motherhood to which women are subjected by society was a theme in her interview. She talked about how so many aspects of being a mother are exposed to society, the world and the family, and are therefore open to scrutiny. This point was very relevant, as Sophia felt she could not hide anymore in the kind of person she was before maternity. Many of her personality traits were also exposed as never before, and she was discovering difficult feelings that she did not display before becoming a mother: anger, loneliness and isolation. She was afraid of being 'submerged' in motherhood to the point of losing her own self. The meaning of the literal word that she used ('submerged') denotes a feeling of being drowned, swamped, immersed or engulfed by the experience. A negotiation was happening in that liminal space of who she was and who she was becoming in the early years of the transition. She articulates this notion in a very clear manner:

> I suppose, before you become a mother, you identify with what you do and it's all about you, you know ... to a certain extent you create yourself ... and what you project to people around you about who you are, 'I'm a yoga teacher, and I do this and I've done that'. You know, this is me, whereas with your kids ... they just arrive with personalities and you can't know what the dynamics are going to be between you and all these different kids, and they're going to ... you know, if you have a few kids, they're all going to press different buttons and bring out parts of yourself that maybe you

were able to keep hidden or present you with challenges that maybe nobody else has ever presented you with ...

Sophia found it was a struggle to find the right balance of being the mother she wanted to be and also fulfilling other parts of who she was.

Innate wisdom: helping and supporting others in the maternal experience

One of the biggest changes that Sophia felt in the transition to motherhood was the way she became more compassionate to other women experiencing difficulties. By the time her first son was three months old, she started looking for a maternal community. She often went to child/parent and breastfeeding meetings. These meetings proved an immense release and support for her. She loved spending time with new mums. The connection she developed with these new mums, and the desire to help other mothers understand what they were experiencing, opened a new role for her. She started training as a pregnancy yoga teacher. During this course, she was able to debrief and face her own experience of birth and all the emotions associated with it that she was still holding on to:

> ... you know, what was a traumatic experience for me has, I think, made me stronger and made me a more compassionate and understanding teacher, and I suppose supporter of women who are pregnant and [have] given birth and breastfeeding ...

Sophia felt that being engaged with the maternal experience, and facilitating others to be so, was part of her own contribution to mothers. Her own reflections on the transition to motherhood emerge from an innate wisdom that she has been trying to connect with and embrace all these years:

> ... new mums ... with lack of self-confidence and insecurity and ... lack of belief in that instinctively, they know how to be mothers. Women tend to be so disconnected from their innate wisdom, their sort of innate wisdom and knowledge that's within them. They can't ... they find it very hard to trust, you know, and to just be. And it's because I've been there and I've sort of come through that and seen my own journey, being very insecure, a sort of slightly in shock new mother to ... I suppose, I've kind of come full circle to being a mum who now helps other mums and it's just so rewarding ...

The connection with that innate wisdom and maternal knowing was crucial to Sophia. In the last part of the interview, she was able to put together the different resources that were helping her to stay connected in her maternal journey. Through yoga, meditation and relaxation practices she has grown an 'awareness of herself'. The importance of these practices is very clear in her narrative:

I did sort of very traditional yoga and through meditation as well and through relaxation practices, so I think I have an awareness of myself and a way of seeing clearly, even if I'm not, even really not always just in the moment, but I can step back and look at situations and look at myself and acknowledge emotions and feeling ... I suppose it helps me connect to my instinct as a mother, to respect it and to honour it. You know, and to be strong ...

Sophia finished the interview by reiterating how self-compassion continues to be the most important practice within herself. The concept of *Ahimsa*,[2] from the Yoga Sutras gives meaning to her experience. She makes a great effort in cultivating an attitude of kindness towards herself. This practice has helped her to accept the unknown and the uncertainties of motherhood.

Sophia read her transcript and wrote a reflection piece. She felt that reading the transcript really helped her to stand back, appreciate who she was, and acknowledge that she was doing her best. She recognised that being in the moment in the maternal experience was very difficult. Her biggest struggle seemed to be her inner critic, whom she continues to challenge. Her attitude was not to cease from exploration: '... I think I will continue to explore and be curious about what motherhood means to me and how I cope with its challenges, like my sense of identity ...'.

Ann: finding a voice through motherhood: maternal blogging

Ann is a mother of three children in her early forties. She has always worked full-time in paid employment. With the birth of her third child, she was finding it increasingly difficult to keep the children 11 hours in a crèche. A whole dichotomy was presented in front of her. Deep feelings, such as regret, resentment, guilt and a sense of failure were common in her mind at that time. One evening she was going home with her husband in the car and a radio programme was talking about the lack of women on company boards and in responsible, managerial jobs. She became angry, as a variety of opinions were being expressed on air, but the real experience of mothers was not. She started texting the radio station. For the first time, she wanted her voice to be heard. She could not hold back anymore. That night, she continued searching for a forum online – a place where maternal voices can be published, heard, owned – even if it is a virtual place. This is how she described the experience:

I wish there was some forum, somewhere you could have conversations like this with other mothers, mothers who work, mothers who want to work, mothers who don't work, but, you know, different kind of situations, it doesn't really matter, just somewhere to have those conversations ...

This is how her blog was born. Ann felt that, instead of calling and shouting at the radio programme, she wanted to have the chance to write. Once the written word is posted, it does not belong to you anymore but to everyone. She was looking for that kind of interaction, away from the isolation of motherhood that she had felt since the birth of her first child. Her blog is one of the most success-ful and widely-read. She often gets to talk on radio shows, when maternal dis-cussions are part of the programmes:

> ... I had a chance to be on a national radio show, one of the days, talking about childcare costs and I was like, 'Oh my God, six months ago I was texting this show and now I'm getting a chance to actually speak on the show'. And that felt like really good, like, *that it was a voice that I had managed to have a voice*, so that was cool' (researcher's emphasis).

Pregnancy and birth: is it really happening to me?

Ann described her first pregnancy with a kind of disbelief. She could not com-prehend the changes in her body, and for her first pregnancy, she was adamant that her life would be the same. Nothing was going to change. She recalled a wedding that she attended when she was seven-months pregnant and how she spent the night dancing away until 2 am. She took pride in the fact that people commented on how the great the way she was handling her pregnancy was, and how she was so tiny – she did not even look pregnant at all. When her water broke at work, she got a book and read about it and then called the hospital. She described herself at that time as clueless. Once she got to the hospital, she was admitted immediately. That night, she sent an email to her boss telling him that she would not be in the next morning.

   The birth of her first child was a shock to her. She recalled not being prepared for the intense pain and wondering if there was something wrong with her and her pain threshold. When her baby was born, she was elated:

> Oh, my God! Like, I don't think there's any way to describe it really, it's just amazing, isn't it? It's just like the most amazing thing and the most mind-blowing thing that you have this person in yours arms who was inside you up to a few minutes previously ...

Her baby was three weeks premature and she felt unprepared to leave the hos-pital and go home. However, after leaving the hospital, she did not recognise the need for postpartum support. A circle of compulsive feeding, weighing and sleeping reduced her life to a minute-by-minute existence. She was losing the notion of time. There was a constant worrying for little daily things, to the point that she was having difficulty keeping any routine:

> Getting her weighed all the time, worrying about feeds: was I feeding her properly. Dealing with the night-time wakings and just trying to figure out how to get dressed, how to get a shower in the morning and now I look back and think, 'Why was that difficult?'.

The realisation of maternity

There was a realisation for Ann that she had no choice and that 'this was her life now'. She felt lonely and isolated. She found her first period of maternity leave really hard:

> You just have to get up every day and do it. Then you would wake up every morning feeling fresh-ish, feeling like, 'OK, we can do this, we can start again'. And by evening time the tears would be there and it would be, you know, waiting for my husband to come home so that I could hand over the baby and have a breather ...

She also started seeing her partner as a functional person who just helped around the house. She described that time as pure survival:

> My husband, to me, just became a person who does stuff in the house. I didn't even see him as a human being anymore, or as my husband or as my partner. I just saw him as the guy who comes home from work and can do stuff that helps me. And I remember that really surreal feeling of that funny attachment that you get to the baby, and it's like you can only be so completely attached to one other human being at a time, so for that early period it was the baby, and therefore I was kind of detached from my husband, so he was there as a functional person who could help me, but not as any kind of a person that I had a relationship with, you know ...

These overwhelming feelings started to subside by the time Ann returned to work. Looking back on the experience, she felt that there was no need for the kind of isolation she endured with her first child. She has written extensively on her blog on those early feelings and the crucial need for networking. All kinds of networking are needed. She encouraged mothers to join maternal groups such as breastfeeding, play, yoga and massages groups:

> It means getting up and out in the morning, which seems impossible: you get to speak to other grown-ups and to share all your problems and, yeah, I just didn't know that, I just stayed in the house when it was. ... Yeah, it was really hard.

The nuclear family versus community

One of the big differences in the twenty-first century is definitely the move from a collectivistic to an individualistic society. This turn has affected the family greatly. Ann is very aware of this shift and the challenges of the nuclear family. Her mum died when she was younger, her sisters work full time and could not help her much and her in-laws live far away. Under these contemporary circumstances, she felt that the mothering experience was hindered:

And it's sad, because it's not supposed to be like that, and I do think, in previous generations it was different, people all lived closer together, nobody would have been left on their own with a new baby to deal with all day every day, sitting at home, or going out on their own to the supermarket, because you need to get out of the house, but you've no one to talk to in the supermarket either, and it just wouldn't have happened in previous generations, and it's sad that that's how we've ended up today and that so many first-time mums don't know that they shouldn't have to deal with everything on their own; and I know it now and I try to pass that message on, but it's going to keep happening, of course it is …

Her own reflection on the transition to motherhood brought her to a conscious change which was based on a 'not-self-centred' experience of herself. Throughout her narrative, she was trying to work out the difficult feelings that emerge in parenting. All feelings are heightened in motherhood. She talked about anger and anxiety and the discovery of a new person that is not so calm. By reflecting on those feelings, Ann came to the conclusion that an acceptance has to happen in order to find any meaning in the experience. Everything mattered more, and the purpose of life seemed to shift in the transition to motherhood. Ann started questioning the desire that brings women to become mothers:

Yeah, I don't know, like I mean, certainly what you do matters more, what the meaning of it all, what the purpose of it all is, I don't know still, even when you think of people saying about when the question comes up: why do we all have kids? I do sometimes think, 'What is the point of all this?'.

These questions, feelings and thoughts were a very isolating experience in Ann's mind. Her transition to motherhood became about making sense and sharing the experience in a wider forum.

Transformation through creativity

Her maternal blog is a form of therapy. By putting her own voice online, she achieved her own transformation of the experience. Her voice started being the voices of so many other mothers. At the end of the interview, when we started talking about her blog, Ann's face lit up. Writing her blog has become her beacon in her maternal transition:

I just love it. I just love it. It's therapy. In my head, I'm already writing down about last night, so if something annoying or bad happens, you write it down and get it out of your head and onto the page or the screen, so that's a therapy in itself. And then, you know, you kind of go, 'Oh, no matter what bad stuff happens, if I can get a blog post out of it, it's something, *it's a silver lining at the end of every challenging experience*'. And then there's that sense of satisfaction when you write something that you're happy with and you press the publish button and it goes out. And then of course it's about the feedback (researcher's emphasis).

Ann is very aware that motherhood has opened a creative path in which she and other mothers can find solace from their own experiences. She recalled the many times she would read, after posting, 'Thank you for writing this'. This constant validation from other mothers creates the need to continue to make an impact. Ann's insight to the transition to motherhood is about flexibility. The maternal experience does not need to be about isolation and stagnation for women. She believes that it is of crucial importance to make sense of the experience by reflecting on the changes that every mother undergoes in the transition. Then, creativity seems to play an important role on how those changes are negotiated. Ann feels that many mothers would like to transform the maternal experience into their lives in a positive way, even if culturally it is difficult.

> ... because employers a lot of the time will only hire people full time, and they don't want to work full time, so I think there are so many mothers in this country who would like to be doing something slightly different and can't, and there's no lobby, no forum, no voice really, so, yeah, I think that's kind of where I'm coming from.

Self-reflection: making sense of the experience

Once Ann had read the transcript of her interview and written her reflection piece, she felt that the experience of telling someone about the transition to motherhood seemed surreal to her. Feelings like regret and disappointment emerged in the reflection piece, especially when reading about the experience of her first child. She kept thinking that she should have managed better at that time. She still feels that she owes something to her eldest daughter for that time.

In the reflection piece, Ann was very adamant that she needed to explain her maternal ambivalence about having children, which she talked about in the interview. Maternal ambivalence is a difficult experience to voice in this culture. An important point she wanted to get across was that 'some people absolutely know they want children'. She could not say for certain that she did not want kids, therefore she guessed she wanted them. Ann feels that nobody is really 'ready' to make such a decision, but the alternative is more frightening to her (leaving it too late and then regretting the decision).

Ann finished her piece with the conviction that making the decision to have children will never lead to regret, and nature is very smart in making mothers love children more than life itself. It is forever impossible to conceive of your life without them, once they have entered it.

Serena: it is a constant and evolving engagement with change

Serena's narrative on her transition to motherhood can be encapsulated in the quotation above. She is in her late 50s and her children are all grown up. She feels that she has gone full circle in the maternal experience. Serena has been involved with mothers for over 25 years in many capacities. During these years, she trained many lactation consultants around the country. She has been mentoring mothers in their transition to motherhood and has recently been conducting workshops on preparing mothers-to-be.

In the interview, she recalled her own transition, but also all that she has learnt during that time from others. Having a child was a very conscious decision. She was 27 years old then. Her circumstances were unusual for the time. She had a very good job so her husband was a stay-at-home dad back in the 1980s.

She described her transition to motherhood as follows:

> The transition to being a mother was the realisation that never again would you make a decision to do something yourself without considering what else had to be done as well. So you couldn't just walk out the door, and do whatever you decided to do. And also, I was a breastfeeding mother. So that added another layer of complication because I also turned out – and I didn't know it at the time, I didn't know what sort of mother I would be – but I turned out to be a very hands-on parent. And that surprised me.

Maternal support: being part of a community

Serena had her children with her all the time – everywhere she went, they went. Her husband brought the children to her workplace at lunchtime and she fed them there. She had no idea what to expect at the time and surprised herself with that notion of a 'hands-on mother'. At the time, this meant that she restructured her whole life around the family. Her career changed, and she began getting involved with maternal and breastfeeding groups and trained to become a breastfeeding counsellor. She described how she was searching for her own philosophy of parenting. When she started associating with other mothers who felt and thought like her, she discovered a community that she could be part of.

She pointed out in her narrative the importance for mothers to find a maternal group that they feel comfortable with. Networking was very important for her then. In her interview, Serena regularly highlighted that it is even more important for mothers to network in these times that when she became a mother back in the 1980s.

Closeness and accessibility: two key points in the transition

Serena was very strong in her opinions, as if she had thought and reflected on the transition to motherhood and its consequences for a long time. One of the crucial points for her was to have her children close to her. This closeness implies not only a physical closeness, but also a deeper access to the mother: 'The meaning of motherhood … I think, I think just being available to be somebody that your children can have access to…'. She recognises how hard is to be available fully if anxiety and loneliness get in the way. She feels how much the world has changed from the 1980s to now, in terms of parenting and the transition to motherhood. Blogging, maternal groups, Facebook forums and other technological resources that she never had in her time are, as she put it, life-savers for a lot of mothers in contemporary society:

> Because I think the mother, you'd need to have *so much reserves to be*, like in yourself, to be able *to keep giving* like that, hour after hour after hour after hour after hour, and you need to be able to have a laugh. Facebook has been a great saviour for lots of women … I see a lot of the girls on Facebook like at 2 o'clock, 3 o'clock in the morning, talking to each other because they're all awake, feeding babies, and it's great (researcher's emphasis).

The importance of laughter in this process is crucial for Serena, otherwise mothers can cry a lot as it is so easy to feel anxious and overwhelmed by the experience. Perfection is one of the signs that she constantly sees while visiting new mothers. Perfection and surveillance have become the two main enemies for the success of this transition. It is interesting to note that, compared to when Serena had her children, these negative feelings are so much more prominent in the twenty-first century:

> I work in the community and I visit mothers and I see mothers, and it's not perfect; when everything isn't perfect, they just feel so sort of shook. They're very shaken by the fact it's turned out not to be perfect, what happens to you, because you continuously fall short so therefore, you doubt yourself.

Doubt and failings seem to be the seeds for an overwhelming transition. These feelings also have the capacity to question the mother to the very core of her abilities and hinder her own maternal identity and self-esteem. Serena has reflected many times on those feelings and came to the conclusion that 'connection' would alleviate some of the pain and pressure that comes with the transition to motherhood.

The importance of inner connection

The kind of connection she talks about in her narrative is the mother's own connection with herself first. The mother needs to know what is happening with her own feelings, worries and stresses, and needs to be consciously honest in order to acknowledge those emotions and be active in helping herself. Serena feels that quality time with herself had been very important in reducing these feelings. A reflective quiet time to gather oneself is paramount. She often teaches mothers that if that intra-connection is not achieved, it will be very difficult to be open and flexible with the following connections needed, for the children and the community in general.

Serena is a very strong, connected person. She still enjoys working for the community of her parish, because it includes people of all ages who enjoy the ritual of being with families for a quiet hour once a week. In a way, her life has been about helping mothers along the way, but not as any parenting guru that we see on television programmes these days. Her contribution has been in helping mothers to know themselves well enough to find their own inner resources. She gets huge satisfaction from being able to entertain and educate at the same time, especially with her mother-to-be workshops. A sense of humour feels very important to her for combating the perfection and pressure that mothers engage with during the transition. The notion of good enough mother versus perfect mother runs through her narrative:

> You just have to be good enough, because if you're striving to be better than that, you would drive yourself nuts. You know, you have to just accept, and also you don't always get the child you bargained for. You've ideas in your head about how your children might turn out and they could be very different. They could be not at all how you thought they might be. Because you look at you and you look at your husband and you think, 'Oh, well, there'll be a bit of each'. But actually, sometimes you get a complete other person who's come with bits from away down the family.

Maternal ambivalence and its difficulties in the transition

Serena is not afraid, in her narrative, to open a dialogue about maternal ambivalence in relation to children. She acknowledges the difficult task that it is to mother a human being who is also an individual and comes to this world with his/her own character. She wants to make clear that the interactions and dynamics in which the mother engages constantly with her children are demanding at many levels. When she speaks about her own children, she considered the differences between them and how to accept them:

> Two of my three children on a fairly regular basis want to kill the third one because he just doesn't … is not motivated to be as helpful as they think he should be, so a bit of warfare has gone on, but I've sort of brought them to a point where I say, 'Look, you've got to accept difference in life, you've got to accept that he isn't you, he doesn't want to be you, he isn't you, leave him be to make his own way and we'll see what he does'.

Serena strongly feels that acceptance, patience and self-kindness need to be cultivated by the mother in order to 'survive' the experience. Motherhood in a contemporary consumer society has been engulfed in a package of illusions to a sanitised, perfect and idealised image:

> They're sold ... they're sold an idea that if you own this buggy, that costly big device, this, that and the other, there's a kind of a myth around mother-hood out there that actually you can do it by numbers, that if you have all the right things, it'll be OK. But *it'll never be OK if you're not OK* (researcher's emphasis).

In talking about new mothers whom Serena has helped through the transition, she emphasises the conviction that it is crucial to handle the disillusionments and transform them into lessons to learn and accept:

> If you actually get stuck in, you are less likely to be disillusioned with it all. I think if you have set the bar very high that you're going to have the perfect house, the perfect partner, the perfect car, life will be perfect and then we'll have the perfect baby. And you get this thing that's wet and squeaky at both ends and hasn't got much to say for himself and controls the household, some people can find that's just an amazingly challenging time to try and get through that.

Negotiating uncertainty, change and the unknown

Much of the feedback that Serena has had from mothers through the years is about how they cannot cope with never knowing what's happening next. It is in this unknown place that a good part of the transition is happening. The liminal time of each individual is a mystery, as every mother is unique. Serena feels that most of the disappointments, deep feelings and also profound transformations happen in this period. It is difficult to measure how long that period will last.

At the stage that Serena is at with her children, she clearly says in her narrative that she has no major regrets. She did not live her life through her children either, but in parallel to them. Still, the most important lesson for her, in the maternal transition, is the constant negotiation and engagement with change.

In reflecting about all the years parenting, she concluded:

> For me, it is very important because it gives you that sense of belonging, of sort of knowing what your role is. And I will never be a mother who will struggle with empty-nest syndrome. Like when my children go, I will be waving them off, because I know I have mothered them and parented them to the best of my ability, so I have no regrets when they flap their little cuckoo wings and leave the nest.

Dana: consider and reconsider constantly the experience and its challenges

Dana is a breastfeeding counsellor, antenatal educator and a doula.[3] She helps mothers to birth and feed their babies and encounters many challenges in this task on a daily basis. She is in her fifties and has four children. Unfortunately, her own transition to motherhood is marked by the death of her own mother. This tragic event impacted her greatly. Her own grief for her mother opened a door for her to reconsider the role of mothers, and how to overcome very difficult situations in this transition. For a long time, Dana could not understand or accept how she lost her mother when she was five months pregnant.

The symbolic 'mother' and grief

In talking about that difficult time, Dana says that she started her maternal work of breastfeeding coach, educator and doula to help women. The mother as an emotional, physical and spiritual 'container' is the presence that Dana tries to recreate for all the women she helps in their transition to motherhood.

She left her job to enter a new career that linked to her need and desire to become a symbolic 'mother' for women. She emphasised how she needed to be with women at that time: 'But, so yeah, I think my desire to be with women, I suppose, and support women is that there is a way that this can happen that you're not feeling destroyed by it [the maternal experience]'. Dana felt that her doula's work brought her the satisfaction to be a maternal 'vessel' for these women. Symbolically, she understood, through the years, that there is a way to go through the experience of birth, and consequently, this transition, without being 'destroyed' by it.

Doula's work: a presence, a touch and a reassurance

The work as a doula helped Dana to recreate a new experience of birth and maternal transition. It has been healing for her to transform her grief into helping others with what she called: 'a presence'. She describes it thus:

> A lot of it is touch and, you know, just being there, physically being there, looking at somebody, just reassuring ... you're supporting them in a way also, but it's all about the woman, it's all about making sure she isn't too frightened, you know, because people get frightened. But I just think it's such a great honour to be asked to be there, you know, to be part of it, such a huge part ... it's like a piece of armour for them, it's like insurance.

This 'motherly' reassurance and presence are what Dana offers in her work. She pointed out that it is all about supporting women in their needs and wishes, not what she thinks is the best thing for them to do.

Fear, worry and guilt: the 'enemies' in the maternal transition

In her own transition, Dana had always struggled with getting and accepting help. She really emphasises now that getting support is crucial in the transition to motherhood. She urges mothers to take the help and stop buying into the cultural 'maternal martyr' archetype in which mothers too often get caught up. It is very interesting to note, in Dana's interview, how she highlights three main 'enemy' feelings in this transition; fear, worry and guilt:

I know certainly for every mother, when you give birth, when that child is handed to you or when you pick up that child first, not only are you picking up that child, but there's a bag of guilt and worry comes with it, you know. And whatever worry you have, when you've resolved that, another one is waiting just to step into its place, because that's what motherhood is. You will constantly worry about them.

Thus, fear, worry and guilt seem to come with the package of the maternal transition. Dana feels that support and help are needed to mediate these intense feelings. She feels that during the transition, it is about managing the expectations that mothers have built while pregnant – especially first-time mothers. They do not have the experience, Dana stressed, and the 'ideal cultural maternal image' does not adjust easily to reality. She found it difficult to ask for help at a time when she needed it most. It is important to note that feelings such as worry, anxiety or fear block the capacity to see beyond them, and most mothers tend to 'endure' in silence or 'get on' with the experience in constant, unnecessary 'suffering'. Dana also talked about how many mothers are having children much later in life: either late 30s or early 40s, and she sees the trend as generating more difficulties for them to 'go with the flow' and adapt to the demanding experience of the transition:

I think because mums are getting older, you know, when they're having their first kids they're older, and they have had this perfect life for so long where they're completely in control of every part of it, down to where 'I'm going to put this here, and it's still going to be there when I come looking for it tomorrow'. You know, it's just such a hard adjustment, you know, we're not as young having children.

Control seems to generate the dichotomy of order versus 'chaos' that children may bring to your life. Dana meets a lot of mothers who are having problems in adjusting to the new life that a baby brings. There is a rush for life to be 'back to normal'. There is also a deep desire and necessity to 'pretend' or assume that the transition will not change any other part of mothers' lives, except that they just have a new member of the family.

Trusting the maternal instinctual knowledge

Dana is convinced that mothers do not trust their own instincts anymore:

> Our mothering instinct is being put into question right from the start, you
> know? It's about them managing their expectations. You know, what did
> you think this was going to be like, what were you expecting? But you hear
> it so often, 'Nobody told us'. And actually I don't believe nobody told most,
> a lot of them, because I know from the antenatal classes and all of the ante-
> natal teachers would say the same, they don't hear, and … they don't know.
> *We don't know what we need to know*, you see. *We've no idea what we need
> to know* (researcher's emphasis).

Dana believes that a different 'knowing' that is not fostered in society or culture
needs to be adopted in order for the mother to 'trust' the experience and make
the necessary changes. Often, she meets mothers 'resisting' the experience and
the challenges that it will bring. The problem with this approach is that we
cannot discriminate what we take out of the maternal experience. She often
encounters how even the joy and the happiness intrinsically present in the
maternal transition may be amiss. If there is a resistance opposing what the
experience brings, there is also a risk of bypassing the good moments that
the transition carries. Sadly, Dana's work is about reassuring the mother that she
needs to navigate this time with the 'knowing' that she will get transformed.
This is the knowledge that she encourages mothers to get 'to know' in
themselves:

> I think what would be great is if mums were encouraged to follow their gut,
> just follow your instinct, what do you think you need to do, what do you
> feel is the best thing to do? We need an expert for everything because you
> couldn't possibly know, how could you know how to look after a baby?

This instinctual maternal knowledge seems to be difficult to trust or even 'listen
to', especially for the new mother. Dana described an 'invisible' connection that
mothers must 'hear' in themselves by the process of self-reflection in this new
experience.

Motherhood as a constant negotiation

Dana is very open about the way in which the various stages of this transition
will challenge the mother's capacity to 'consider' and 'reconsider' how to negotiate the different times of the experience. She herself is at the stage where two
of her children are entering puberty. It is a difficult time and many new capacities are needed to 'survive' the many challenges encountered:

> Oh my God! And I stop myself because I don't want to wish away these
> years, but I'd love just a little glimpse that we're there and it's all OK,

they've all survived it. How do you manage to breathe in the meantime 'til they come back or until you get the phone call? I suppose that's where the trust comes in. That's what I have to keep saying, that please God, we have done, we've taught them enough that they will survive and that they won't do stupid things. And yet you know they're going to do stupid things, but hopefully they'll be safe stupid things.

The 'unknown' plays an important role in this process. As Dana points out, often the mother does not know how things are going to play out. A constant trust is necessary to get through the different stages of the transition, even when doubt and mistrust enter the mother's mind. This negotiation is crucial in the maternal transition. The mother's ability to mediate all of the feelings that come with uncertainty from the very beginning of this experience will relieve the 'suffering' that comes with 'not knowing' the future. Living in the now, with the persistent emotions that these stages create, can be very draining. Children live in the now, as the past and the future do not enter their experiences. Living in the now with them is one of the experiences that Dana feels is more difficult to negotiate for new mothers.

Control, anxiety, fear, worry and guilt will hinder this process. She sees that there is a tendency to 'fight' these feelings as mothers can feel so vulnerable and tired. This tiredness can be physical as well as emotional. This is where the self-reflection comes into play. A mother needs to listen and trust that 'instinctual voice' in herself that will help her to go into the unknown of these many stages in motherhood. It is an ongoing process. It is the realisation that going with the unknown is not dangerous, but that it will open more possibilities for the mother to grow and connect with her children and, ultimately, herself. Openness and flexibility are important qualities to foster in the transition. Dana trusts that the current experience will bring her to another place she does not know, and so she is open and trusting in it:

Your gut is going to tell you. Because we all have a conscience and if we listen to our conscience, maybe we're not doing our best, but if we're not getting that little niggling gnawing doubt in our minds, which I know a lot of people do anyway ... I haven't got a clue. And I know we'll survive it.

In her reflection piece, Dana notes that she read the whole transcript of her interview. She could not read the entire piece together, as she felt so emotional re-encountering her experience. The connection and the loss of her mother impacted her in such a way that she feels her own maternal transition has been heavily influenced by it.

Early in the interview, I asked her the question: what do you really think that a woman needs when she is in labour, when she is giving birth? Her response caught me by surprise, as it was such a definitive one. Dana did not even have to think about it. She immediately said: 'her mother'.

Eve: if you go to battle, you have to soldier

Eve is in her early fifties and has three children. She comes from a large family of eight siblings and she is the youngest. Her family culture was very important to her and it was clear from the very beginning of her transition that she was going to do what she had learned in her own family. The culture of her family, and how they looked after babies, was crucial for her and it provided a container for her once she became a first-time mother. She remembered how difficult it was making the early decisions once the baby was handed back to her. Feeding and separation were the main things she was determined to do as her own family had taught her. She had a deep desire to breastfeed, and it was very difficult for her at the beginning:

> I'm breastfeeding this baby and that's it. And I did eventually manage to get going, but it was hard. It was easy on the girls but it took me, just the latching on … I was determined because my own family, all my sisters had breastfed their children.

Her struggle regarding whether to go back to work or stay with her baby was also easy enough to resolve, because her mother and father looked after her first baby. Looking back with 16 years of parental experience, she feels that was the right decision. It was very challenging for her to leave the baby in a crèche. The emotional and physical connections she felt in the transition to motherhood were overwhelming, and she reached for her family of origin and the 'maternal cocoon'. Eve lives within walking distance of many members of her family and it was a 'life- saver' for her in this transition. It is interesting to note how the urban culture of a nuclear family did not affect her, and she often talked of the many benefits she experienced by having her own family as a nearby community, and what a support they were to her in the maternal transition: 'For me personally, because I'm a complete softy, I have the emotional thing about would he be looked after. I was lucky that my parents wanted to mind him'.

Breastfeeding: maternal connection in the transition

For Eve, breastfeeding provided the container for her maternal transition. She feels that breastfeeding contributed to her wellbeing and helped her to negotiate many aspects of being a new mother:

> The connection, well I think the breastfeeding first is a real starting point, because you can't pass your baby over, you can't. Now with M, I only fed him until I went back to work, with the girls I fed them until they were a year. And then that finished, so that's the first thing, that physical connection through breastfeeding.

Breastfeeding became a 'time out' with her babies, where it seemed time stood still; it was just the mother and the baby. It is an intense, embodied connection, but Eve believes that it was a natural way for her to ease into motherhood. It did not come without its challenges, but Eve thought it important to persevere until her breastfeeding routine was established:

> I was a very anxious mother about breastfeeding, because I didn't want bottles. I went in very determined. And it worked because actually they told me after a few days, maybe you should give him a bottle, I said, no, no, no, I'm breastfeeding this baby and that's it. And I did eventually manage to get going, but it was hard. Some mothers would say it wasn't difficult to get it started, I had a nurse coming in doing this and doing that and doing this with his mouth and oh my God, but I was really determined to.

Eve felt that from the very beginning she needed to trust some maternal instincts that were being put into question inside herself. This trust pivoted on the ability to breastfeed her baby, and how important it was for her. Success in this aspect would have been crucial for her confidence in her own abilities to 'mother' in the way that was important for her. Family culture played an essential role in her decisions.

Trusting her own body and abilities came with anxiety for the baby. She recalled how she would ask for the baby to be weighed, to make sure that he was thriving:

> It wasn't enough for me to have a nurse come to weigh him: I asked for the consultant paediatrician to come and weigh my baby. I mean, ridiculous, you know, I mean, but they were so lovely. She had seen him and she said, if you're concerned and you want him weighed again, come back. And I went back and the nurse said, we'll weigh him, and I said, oh no, I'd like to see the doctor.

These unrealistic demands seem absurd now to Eve, but she can remember how vulnerable she felt after the birth. This vulnerability puts the new mother at a certain risk, as she cannot respond in the same way as she would under normal circumstances. She felt that the members of the hospital, family and friends were crucial for support during this period. She was very open to admit how easy it is to follow the anxiety created by the 'unknown' in this transition, and how difficult it is to recover from it after it happens.

Support network in the maternal transition

Eve recalled how friends are so important in helping the new mother. The isolation of motherhood and the belief, as she calls it, of 'doing the wrong thing', can dissipate if the support network is there for the new mother: 'There's no one to teach you, you're learning as you go along, that's how our mothers learned and before them and before them. But of course, I did seek advice'. Seeking advice of friends or family broke the anxiety for Eve, and she often shared her worries with more experienced mothers:

> I have a very close friend who has six children, and she was one person I used to phone. How long do you think she should sleep, do you think that, yeah, she was a great one for just back up, you know, yeah. But just naturally you're wondering are you doing it right.

Eve felt that, naturally, mothers are always wondering and aiming for some kind of perfection that has no end. It was an act of empowerment to have people around her for validation on how she was doing in her own maternal transition. In a sense, it could be said that it is not the advice that helps mothers, but the constant support and validation on how they are managing different situations.

Parenting challenges: how children teach parents to grow

Eve encountered a bigger challenge with her second child as she had a learning disability:

> My second child has a learning disability, so that was harder to cope with. She's 14 now and she's in a special school down the road and she's a great girl and she really is super, but that whole having to deal with that, was very challenging. And we knew from about the time she was one, because she was a floppy baby, she couldn't sit up, she couldn't crawl and she didn't walk until she was nearly four.

Eve admits not only how challenging this situation can be, but how it opens a place in the mother to change and adapt in a very different way. She had to learn patience, compassion and understanding on a new level. She needed to live in the present on a daily basis and negotiate her own expectations.

> I look back, I met so many lovely other parents and families that I'm still friendly with, and the therapists, the therapists who were so supportive. It was challenging but our motto is we live for today and next week and the next month, but you don't start racing ahead.

Eve believes that the personality of the mother interplays with her children's personalities. How capable the mother is in managing the intertwining of personalities is crucial for the success of the transition. She has to learn how to cope by responding to her challenges and change according to what it is going to be best for the family. This requires a lot of effort on the mother's part. Children highlight many parts of the mother's personality that need certain growth and change, and it is the ability to accommodate these changes, without any drama, that is important:

I think just our own personalities, it's what, it's how we are, isn't it? Our own disposition. I hope never to get caught up in over ... wanting so much more than they're capable of. But all we all want, isn't it true, is for our kids to be the best they can be?

Having a child with a learning disability has changed the whole family, and what they had to learn opened a door for them to be better in themselves. Eve has managed to convert challenges into advantages by learning and being open to the experience. It has become an enriching experience:

For the whole family but specifically them as children, they don't even realise what they're learning, all the attributes of *patience, compassion, understanding.* Also, our world is filled – our family world and our friend-ships – with individuals who have learning disabilities (researcher's emphasis).

This highlights the difference in how to approach the unknown in parenting and the unknown in the transition to motherhood. Eve is very strong in her interview, showing her focus is not on the challenges, worries and anxieties that can be brought by this transition, but the way mothers respond to them. Networking and family support were crucial for her. Her own husband is a rock for her, as she described:

I've a great husband: a united front. He's a great dad, he's a very, very funny person, very, very strong sense of humour, always joking, never walks in the door without, I'm home, and a big happy smile. And not every-thing's great in work, but he's a very positive person. And so for me yes, the love of my own family and all that enrichment that comes with just being loved and knowing that you are loved, and then my own marriage is my absolute sacred belonging, no one else, you know, that's very important.

Eve showed in her words how a 'united front' is paramount for her in order to parent. She recalled the many changes that the couple undergo when they become parents, but it is that union that will keep everything together:

All of a sudden overnight you can't walk out the door without a child on your shoulder or in buggy but just the sheer responsibility of not just being you and your husband anymore. We just went out and, also your money had to be spent differently. Financially you had to accommodate another little person in your family circle and then a second and then a third.

Love, stability and security: how to mediate the transition

For Eve, two main things assisted her in the transition to motherhood. They are all very tightly related to her family of origin and the family she has created. The first one was the love she felt from her own family background that helped her to replicate the same conditions for her family and herself. Her experience showed that a mother's family background can influence her greatly in the ability to recreate such a safe and secure position for the family and for herself. She is convinced that she would have been a different person if she had not had such a secure family. The second one was her own positive connection with her mother, and how this facilitated how confident she felt in mothering her own children.

> Oh yes, love of my own family, and specifically that would be coming from my parents, so I came from a very contented, happy family background. That's not everybody's story. I would be a different person today. I've always had stability. Very secure, so the security and the love of family I think would have been one of the most determining factors as to why I think I've done a pretty good job with my own children. Yeah, am I similar to the way my mother? I think yeah, probably.

Her mother once told her, 'if you go to battle, you have to soldier', but Eve remembered she was never judgemental. She was always a container and an encouragement in her own transition to motherhood: 'Oh my goodness, my mother was fantastic, she was great, she was wonderful with babies and never told me what to do. No, because she knew I was learning'.

Clare: listen to all those internal messages

Clare is 46 years old and has three children. She got married at 30 and she remembered how quickly she got pregnant. She was expecting her first child after her honeymoon. Reflecting on her own transition to motherhood, she was very clear on how the process had changed her:

> I didn't realise how much independence you lose, how it changes you, you know that you have to kind of just abandon it, you know, you don't have to kind of go … you know the proper transition is when you stop trying to be the person that you used to be and you just accept the fact I am a mother now and then it is easy.

It has probably taken her 16 years to summarise the meaning of this transition, but she is very convinced of the fact that the key to success is stopping fighting 'the person that used to be'. Every transition has many shocks to overcome when changing is happening at all levels. Acceptance seems to be the crucial point for Clare to comprehend and assimilate her own transition. She faced several challenges in her own transition.

How to embrace the transition and its consequences

Clare used the word 'embrace' to describe this transition. She pointed out how contemporary culture does not facilitate the change. Instead of facilitating the change, the language around the maternal transition is about 'getting back to the way the mother was before having the baby'. Clare feels that this cultural dimension is experienced at various levels, including the emotional, social, economic and certainly the physical (the mother's body):

> This whole thing about getting back in to your jeans and getting back out there and everything, that is the piece that is hard. You have to accept – no this is you now there are other parts of me now, *there is a dependency* and you can't just … so this whole – I think there is a whole drive for, you know, get back in your jeans, get out there, go out with the girls, put them in a crèche, have them sleeping all night, they are grand, they are grand, they are grand, it is all about … (researcher's emphasis).

Clare realised that she was not ready for the 'dependency' that comes with the transition. She needed to learn a lot about herself and about her baby, in order to balance the enormous dependency that is felt during this process. Babies come full of dependency and needs, and these interact with the mother's own dependency and needs, and all of the aspects in her life. Leaving her baby was particularly difficult for Clare. Her maternity leave finished and she had to be separated from the baby:

> I had a good job. I did a lot of travelling. I did a lot of business travelling. I used to fly to London once a week and I used to fly to Berlin once a week. The hard thing was going back to work. I had to go back to work when he was four and a half months old. It was horrible.

It was at this time that Clare started to feel she was getting mixed messages from society, friends and family. It was the beginning of her transition, and she was not confident enough to decide on what was best. Feeding, sleeping, separation, connection, stay at home versus going to paid work, all became issues that she had to face. She remembered getting a book from the library about parenting from the seventeenth century to the present day. It was a revelation to her how people have parented through the centuries. The transition to motherhood changed accordingly to the needs of the times people were living in:

> This was a book that summarised all the different baby theories from seventeenth century to modern times. When you look back, the kind of parenting that was recommended reflected a society at the time; 50 percent of babies died up till 1920 or 1930. It didn't really matter what was recommended, because no matter what you did, they died. So, you know, they would wrap them up and hang them up on a hook to keep them off the floor. Nobody knew what was working and what wasn't working. Then in the First and

Second World War about not attaching because you were rearing them for war. And put them outside and crying exercises the lungs and everything and people at that time were trying to do the best for their children.

By reflecting on this information, Clare started to trust more what she thought was the best for her baby, instead of listening to the current culture. Clare began to experiment with an intense feeling of 'going with her gut', in the process of maternity. She distinguished the intellectual, rational knowledge with a different knowledge that she was trying to reach into: 'I knew intellectually, you know, one person is telling you this and one person is telling you that. I just said, 'no I am not following those rules. I am going to go with my instincts'. Going with her instinctual knowledge meant that Clare was trying to reconcile the enormous dependency with her internal resources, and how to negotiate the needs of the baby and also her own needs. Her decisions from then on were about building a deep connection between the baby and herself. Metaphorically, she called this connection a 'bank', in terms of how emotional transactions were made in this process:

> I suppose you know to allow yourself to respond to your instincts with your children. It is often what your body or your gut tells you. You are giving them attention and you are giving them the comfort that they need, it is all going into the bank you know, both banks. Completely connected but if you are that connected and the satisfaction and the joy and the reward back is so strong.

Clare feels that the mother needs to foster that self-connection first, and then with the baby. Connections are difficult and it is a multifactorial process. Being connected implies not only the physical and emotional, but also the instinctual. It is hard to live in the present moment and, as Clare puts it in her interview, 'the old person in the past is over, and fighting it will not bring the old life back'. That connection is a kind of presence that serves as self-container and baby container, simultaneously. It requires letting go and an 'embracement' of the new self:

> I would say just allow yourself to do it and I know it is short, you know, they say the days are long and the years are short. Because look at me now: the kids are in the house and nobody is calling for me.

The realisation of a new reality within the transition can seem endless while it is happening, but Clare felt that the baby years are not that long, and that 'banking' the trust and the connection can reap rewards in the future. It was crucial for her to listen to those internal messages.

Trusting the maternal knowing

Clare wanted to trust the maternal knowing by listening and reflecting on her own interactions with the baby and herself in the transition. In order to see the whole picture, she relied on her own trust to go with the process and its challenges:

> You see it is not, but if you try and do it intellectually, you don't get the answer because you are ignoring too much information, you know, it is about that. Trusting your own self yeah, yeah trust yourself to learn it, you know. But it was great, one of the most powerful things that happened to me.

There are many decisions in this transition that will challenge the mother's psychosocial world, and as many mothers before her, Clare faced the challenge of her career being disrupted in the process:

> I detached. It didn't feel that important. It just felt like it was work to do but it wasn't all embracing and all-encompassing, whereas previously I would have been 'this is really important' you know like the whole thing whereas, yes, my focus changed and I think that is something that happens to people when they have children.

Her priorities changed, and she described how her value system, which was important for her family life, also underwent a big shift. She found it difficult to make the decision to work part time, but she was sure that the corporate culture did not suit her needs at that time:

> What I am saying is, because I was absorbed by my baby, I felt like I had this new insight really, that I wasn't buying into that whole corporate culture to the same extent. Actually, there was a huge transition at work. A lot of adjustments. But I felt quite, you know, I was used to being professional and being successful and good decision-maker and being in control and things working out for me when I made decisions – things working out for me. My relationship with him [my baby] and him with me and how he was doing, but also interactions felt important.

Clare found that it was difficult to build a career after being out of work for so long in the corporate world. Reconciling family and work was difficult and she felt that the dichotomy of becoming a mother and being in a corporate job was put to her in a very real way. Her own self-reflection about her new life brought her to make the best decision she felt for her family. She had three children under five years old at the time.

Clare started to rely more on the support network, such as parenting organisations and other mothers in the same situation. She felt that she needed to get out of the house and be involved in activities with the children. The importance of a support system was a 'saver' to her in her 'self-constructed mothering':

> That's for me I needed the people who came with the new life. You know whereas at work, you interact with your colleagues and you might like them or not but they are just people you interact with because this is what you are doing; so it is the same I needed that.

The future: the decisions that the mother makes in the transition

Once life-changing decisions are made in one's life, they need to serve a tangible purpose in the future. Clare felt that the different decisions she made along the way gave her the satisfaction she expected of them. Now that she has a teenage son, she relies on the connection she built through the years. Clare has noticed that it is easier for her to reach her son because the amount of work she has done:

> I suppose it is a sort of lean in thing, you know, reach in to that connection and lean in because the more connected you are with them. I still would have very strong connections with my oldest son. I would be well able to say to him you know 'how's it going?'.

Clare's transition is marked by her determination to listen to her internal messages and build her own trust. She reflected on the culture and the storied tradition of motherhood. She embraced her own self-constructed motherhood and found meaning and solace in the deep understanding of her interactions with her children and herself. She relied on instinctual knowledge by asserting her own trust and maternal authority. Those resources were paramount in how Clare negotiated her transition, and she summed it up at the end of her interview as follows: 'You would lose a lot by not going with your gut. You know, because really what makes us feel alive is the human interactions, you know'.

Barbara: the loss of identity in the maternal transition

Barbara's transition to motherhood was very difficult. She was 27 years old when she got pregnant and she felt too inexperienced to have a baby. At the time, in the 1980s, she was working as a journalist and a researcher. She started seriously thinking about an abortion, but recalled how her sister-in-law told her mother, and it was nearly impossible to go ahead with it. Barbara blamed the sex education system and the whole culture in which she was brought up:

> My mother would not let her three daughters use tampons. My middle sister disobeyed her but I was too frightened of disapproval. As a couple, we were often in bed together but were terrified to attempt sex over the eight years we dated. I got pregnant "miraculously" when our fumbling around in a

freezing apartment led to an unplanned pregnancy. We felt we were having a baby without even having had sex.

She did not feel ready to get married and motherhood:

> I think I wasn't ready for motherhood I think from my own background really, I had very little experience of looking after babies. It all became very rushed but I think there was a huge relief when we decided we will get married and we will have this baby and we will live at home with my mother and father because we would have no money.

When Barbara got married, tragedy befell her family. The day after her wedding, her mother went into a psychiatric hospital having had a nervous breakdown. She felt that because she was the youngest in the family, her mother could not cope with losing her. Barbara's mother had already had two major losses in the family. Barbara's brother died when he was 16 of a heart attack, while playing rugby, and seven years later, her middle sister killed herself.

By the time Barbara was ready to have her baby, she realised that she had no parents to rely on. Her father was an invalid and her mother was diagnosed with bipolar disorder. These events were to greatly mark her transition to motherhood.

The birth and the loss of her identity

Barbara missed her mother and the support she could have provided in the transition to becoming a mother. The birth and labour were a good experience for her, however, and she remembered the immense joy that overwhelmed her hours after having the baby:

> The birth was so much better and then everything was just getting better and better and better and then I couldn't work out why everybody else was miserable. Then I remember feeling very creative after the birth, I wanted to write, you know, because I did history, then I did journalism and I love to write and then they wouldn't let me have any paper because they said it just mad, you know, I wasn't sleeping because I was so excited and I was just high, high, high.

Barbara had a rush of creativity after birth. Psychiatrists felt that she was in a manic state and they decided to internalise her into a psychiatric hospital until she had recovered a better sense of herself:

> I hadn't expected to love this little creature, this amazing creature. The psychiatrist, you know, comes in and says, 'You have to go to hospital from here, you can't go home with your baby'. I still thought everybody is just exaggerating, everybody has made a mistake, everyone, you know, this will sort itself out, you know, they are all being over cautious.

Barbara recalled being emotionally and physically shut down in the hospital. She spent six months there. Family used to bring her baby once a week, while she felt completely disconnected from everything. It took her almost a year to regain any sense of self. She felt completely unprepared for motherhood and unable to care for a baby. She felt everyone was better at it than her. An event occurred at home when her little girl was barely a year old that shifted the way she thought about mothering:

> I remember we were sitting on a sofa myself and my husband in this rented house and Megan[4] was kind of late learning to walk and she was walking towards us and she fell and she started to cry and she got up and she came to me. At that moment I felt she wants me, she wants me. She came to me.

This major event for Barbara started a new road in her own transition. She felt equal to her husband, which she did not feel before. She regained her confidence that she could mother and, most importantly, she was assured that she had her baby's love.

Finding a place of solace: parental networking

When Barbara moved to a new house, she found a parental organisation through a neighbour. She received visits and phone calls to help her with her feelings in motherhood. She was also invited to mother groups to share her experience. It was a breakthrough out of her isolation:

> It was just wonderful. I felt that I found my place and that I wasn't a strange person, you know, I had felt such a failure as a mother, you know. You don't have equal relationships with people anymore, the stigma of that breakdown. But you can go to a mothers group and everybody is equal.

The support of maternal groups was paramount in Barbara's recovery:

> It was an opportunity to be in a supportive environment that cared about me as an individual and wanted me to be whole again, instead of a broken creature. They could sense my pain and were a vital element in putting back some of the pieces in my destroyed psyche. There were no miracles. Many negative bad habits remained from childhood where my high expectations of myself were matched by even higher levels of insecurity, doubt and self-loathing.

Barbara not only wanted to share her experiences, but she also wanted to help other mothers who may have had postnatal depression. At the time, there was no consciousness about that kind of depression, and Barbara felt like she was on a 'crusade' to educate and contribute to the awareness of it. She got involved in pre- and postnatal groups and wrote articles in national newspapers about the experience of postnatal depression. She was beginning to feel stronger and wanted to 'voice' and recuperate what she felt it was taking from her:

> No I wasn't feeling shameful. Yes, to give myself identity again. That joy of motherhood was stripped away from me by them because I hadn't expected that joy of motherhood and they took it away from me for six months in hospital and then I had to work, work, work to regain that.

Barbara was determined to change how the system treated mothers with this condition. With her second baby, she felt more prepared to deal with all the feelings and bodily experiences that came back once again:

> On day three, the same happened, so it was incredible. It was like a wave; it was like a tsunami. You feel as if you could see it coming because you could almost feel a vibration. It was so powerful and so physical for me. I acknowledge that this illness is hitting me again and I accept that I will have to go to hospital but the promise was to go to what they called the mother and baby unit.

Barbara met four mothers with postnatal depression in the same unit with their babies. She realised that there was a need to be aware of this condition. This second time around, she only spent two days in hospital and then went home for the rest of the week.

In the end, Barbara felt she wanted to write a book on postnatal depression and be involved in helping mothers. This cause, as she described it in the interview, became her passion.

Experiential help: creating a space for other mothers

After listening to many mothers in groups, Barbara realised that she was lucky. Her experiences were extreme, so she had the opportunity to be treated. She realised that other mothers, who did not fit the postnatal depression criteria, did not get any help: 'I used to think well I've had the worst experience possible but when I have talked to other mothers they said, "Well no I've had maybe one year or two years of misery at home, empty, unloved"'. There was very little research into motherhood studies at that time. Maternal anxiety, and other conditions that are not classified as psychiatric disorders, were not considered important enough to warrant treatment. Barbara realised that many mothers whom she had met were struggling in silence in the transition to motherhood. Culturally, they were supposed to cope naturally, but that was far from fact. In maternal groups, Barbara began to listen to statements such as: 'No one took any notice of my despair or my distress'. She also received many letters from women who had read her articles in the paper: 'I got all these letters from women who had never had another baby, you know, from the 1960s, 1970s, they never had another baby because they were so scared'. Her passion to support mothers in the transition to motherhood grew. She cofounded a parental organisation, ran maternal groups and attended many committees to politicise the issue of helping mothers through this transition. She felt she wanted to change the world, but her own insecurities returned to her. At the verge of creating a different experience for other mothers and herself, Barbara always seemed to come to a painful place. In her interview, she mentioned she felt destroyed by the system many times. It has been hard for her to let go:

> I often worked for free and I think one of the huge things for working for free was feeling that I wasn't good enough to be paid. I'd lost my confidence. It's very hard to feel a good person again. I don't know. I worked for free for politicians but it's very disappointing when you work and work for free and you kind of hope that maybe that will lead to a paid job but it never did. I don't know whether that was my fault. You see the problem is that I was diagnosed with puerperal psychosis after each child, so that's the worst end of postnatal depression.

How to regain the sense of identity

Barbara has worked hard in order to regain an identity that she felt she had lost in becoming a mother. Her own background was hard for her, but her experiences in the maternal psychiatric units seemed to have marked her life. She co-wrote a book on postnatal depression. This was a big project for her, and it meant that she could show her concrete experiences and use them in helping others. She recalled being on a 'high' while writing the book. The day the book was launched, she felt great satisfaction for her achievements.

After many years, Barbara was feeling exhausted from her own 'crusade', and could no longer go on with a cause that she felt had given her a sense of a new identity:

> Again it was a case of having high expectations. I hoped that by working on that cause, it would make me closer to my old self. It involved my old skills of writing, campaigning and intellect. I still had *huge expectations of fame and fortune but without the foundations of a grounding balanced psyche.* I was single-handedly going to change the system, whilst being unable to cope with any degree of criticism (researcher's emphasis).

Barbara has now felt more grounded for a number of years. Her psychiatrist organised a weekly mindfulness course as an outpatient in the hospital. This practise has proven very beneficial and now Barbara lives life with more joy. Her feelings of failure and disappointment are slowly disappearing with her mindfulness practice.

On reflecting on her transition to motherhood, she concluded:

> Mindfulness brings joy, like motherhood brings joy. Motherhood also brings anxiety and hurt, and loving and hating, and ignorance and mistakes and success. It is a wondrous challenge and a huge privilege. I am blessed with two amazing daughters who are a credit to their parents.

Notes

1 Names have been replaced with pseudonyms.
2 Ahimsa in Buddhist tradition is a term meaning not to injure, and compassion. It is a multidimensional concept inspired by the fact that all living beings have the spark of the divine spiritual energy; therefore, to hurt another being is to hurt oneself.
3 A woman who gives support, help, and advice to another woman during pregnancy and during and after the birth.
4 Names of children have been changed.

Part IV

Motherhood and spiritual care

8 Uncovering the maternal transition
Prenatal, birth and postnatal experiences

There is always a duality operating in motherhood discourses (paid working mums versus stay-at-home mums, breastfeeding versus bottle feeding, etc.) and understanding the identity of mothering. The task in this discussion is to tolerate opposing forces (Esbjorn 2003), to present the maternal experience with all its complexities and to avoid a 'black and white' framework.

A transition is a threshold that is marked by three points in time and space: (1) pre-transition; (2) 'passing', 'birth' or 'liminal space'; and (3) post-transition. In the transition to motherhood, prenatal, natal and postnatal experiences are those three points in time and space. These temporal three points of the transition are used to present the various themes and trends that emerged out of the mothers' interviews. Themes as connections and change/transformation are part of various points in the transition. These themes are called trans-temporal themes, as they appeared through the three temporal points of the maternal transition.

Pre-transition: prenatal experiences

Prenatal experiences were the experiences that all seven mothers spoke least about. In the interviews, it was difficult to have them recall or go back far enough to remember what they were feeling and experiencing at that time. All seven mothers spent a few minutes talking about their lives 'before' becoming a mother, and then they wanted to move on to discuss birth and postnatal experiences. This type of response can be a direct consequence of the nature of a transition in itself. So many changes happen at various levels in the individual during a transition that it may be hard to remember the times of pre-transition. The main themes/trends to be analysed in the pre-transition period are limited to the desires, expectations and illusions that facilitated and sometimes hindered entering into the maternal transition. The role of spirituality in mediating this first phase, and also the spiritual capacities that mothers utilised in their initial decision to become a mother, are discussed.

Desire, expectations, illusions: their spiritual meaning

All mothers talked about the desire to have children and how they felt at the pre-transition stage. This desire is complex in how it is understood by society. Their responses seem to vary between physical, emotional and unconscious urges. Very few studies have investigated the nature of the desire for women to become a mother. Montgomery *et al.* (2010, 55) concluded that some of the complex factors that lead to a woman's desire to become pregnant are 'the intersection of wanting, personal priorities, and life circumstances'. Issues such as timing, meeting personal criteria and desire for the experiences of pregnancy, birth and parenting, were also very strong factors in the decision to have a child.

There is often a sort of tension between socially-controlled fertility and fertility controlled by the individual or couple. Research has demonstrated that social and cultural learning frequently impacts on women's desire for reproduction (Bongaarts and Watkins 1996; Kohler 2001). Some mothers viewed having children as something that would happen at some point in their lives. As they were all in relationships, the desire to have children was a 'natural' course of their love. Reproduction has been described as 'culturally naturalised' (Ravn 2005). Having children cannot, therefore, be construed as a choice at all in these circumstances, as it is simply something that is supposed to happen at some point in a couple's life together.

Some researchers argue that women are not 'naturally' or 'essentially' mothers. Instead of being instinctual, motherhood for many women may depend on the environment, and the individual circumstances in which each woman finds herself' (Hrdy 1999; Liesen 2001). Today there may be many objectives that women desire to accomplish before becoming pregnant or making personal decisions about the pregnancy. In contemporary Western society, most women want to be in a secure financial situation, have a stable partner, have travelled, held a successful career and be a suitable maternal age before considering pregnancy. Many studies corroborate these realities (Benzies 2008; Benzies *et al.* 2006; Romo *et al.* 2004). Some psychoanalysts believe that the motivation to become a mother is often accompanied by an unconscious wish to release archaic raptures, to retrieve and rework undigested experiences or heal early scars (Raphael-Leff 2003, 57).

Some mothers discussed a 'body urge' as a reason for having a baby. Most women are somewhat conscious of their body's potential to give birth from childhood. Therefore, from the beginning, women need to take some kind of stance regarding this potential. The problem with such a 'natural choice' approach is that the women may end up bearing sole responsibility for the child. It has been argued that if motherhood is seen exclusively as an individual woman's personal response to an urge, there is no need to improve parental rights in the labour market (Sevon 2005). This argument is very significant and complex. Women can be 'penalised' in society for their own desires for reproduction. Women's desire to reproduce is thus intrinsically related to the female body. Even though giving birth is not an absolute necessity for a woman, motherhood philosophy is often firmly grounded within female embodiment (Battersby 1998).

Studies demonstrate that unconscious and conscious factors are usually collectively in operation in maternal decision-making. The desire for mothering, as well as for refusing mothering, may emerge in embodied subjects from memories and cultural narratives; from unconscious and conscious identifications (and refusals to identify) with representations of motherhood (Kaskisaari 1999). Therefore, this desire is a 'lived experience' that has deep unconscious habits and thus is not fully rationally explicable. It is a transition which is embodied, and unconscious, and thus haphazard and unforeseeable (Sevon 2005).

There is a connection between the desire for reproduction and spirituality. Life with children is perceived by many in this study to represent something fundamental for existence itself. All participants in this study described having children as giving deep meaning to their lives. This 'deeper meaning' transcends beyond the mother's own individuality, thus transforming her own identity (Ravn 2005). All mothers seemed to construct personal meaning within the desire to become a mother. It is within this transformation that most of postnatal experiences were also accounted for in this study.

The desires and the effect are directly related. Mothers will experience social capital, new social connections and deep identity change in the transition to motherhood. Thus, the main spiritual capacities that may be mediated by entering the transition are: meaning-production, 'embodied knowing' and a more conscious awareness of personal identity.

Entering this transition can be described as both a conscious and an unconscious embodied spiritual call, similar in character to the classical experience of vocation. All mothers in this study were the biological mothers of their children and, thus, their desire for reproduction marked the self's 'spiritual knowing' with the experience of the 'embodied knowing' (Parratt 2010). This type of 'spiritual knowing' is the life-meaning that mothers in this study attached to having children and becoming mothers. Six of them asserted that their decisions were conscious, although it is important to note that one mother expressed ambivalence in relation to her decision in becoming a mother. Human desire and intentions are of vital importance in comprehending the interaction between the human mind, the psyche and the spirit. The human spirit has an unconscious dimension in which these desires, intentions, expectations and motivations reside (Helminiak 1996; Perrin 2007). To be able to conceptualise the role of how spirituality impacts on the beginning of the transition to motherhood is to recognise the incorporation of the 'lower dynamics' (psyche) into the 'higher dynamics' (spirit), with the collaboration of the thinking mind.

Illusion is defined as 'an erroneous perception of concept, belief or reality'.[1] Expectation is defined as 'a strong belief that something will happen or be the case in the future'.[2] If expectations and illusions are combined in the woman's mind, it can create a 'maternal parallel reality' that seems to serve as a form of solace during the prelude to the transition. Most expectations are idealised in the mother's psyche. But becoming a mother involves moving from a known, current reality to an unknown, new reality (Mercer 2004). By reviewing one transcript of a mother's interview, the collaboration of the psyche, mind and spirit can be elucidated:

> When I was pregnant, I imagined I was going to do things a certain way, everything will be just as I want it to be. I am a calm and organised person. I read an autobiography and the main character is described as an earth mother. She takes her three beautiful daughters, all lovely, dressed for a picnic, and I remember thinking: '*I want this*'. We'd just go off on adventures and head off in the car, and have such great fun and, you know we'd all just be so happy and I do yoga so my kids will be so calm and blah, blah, blah (researcher's emphasis).

> (Sophia's transcript)

In the above transcript, this mother is envisioning an idealised picture of motherhood, which she desires. By visualising this idyllic picture of the earth mother with her daughters on a picnic, she is not afraid to enter the transition, and she is sure that she has the resources for it. The earth mother may function as a positive maternal archetype which, spiritually, mothers can aim to be like. Psychological positive expectations about motherhood have been correlated with positive adjustment to the role, while negative expectations have been associated with poorer adjustment (Kach and McGhee 1982; Wylie 1979). Such positive expectations, although unrealistic, may be compared to individuals in romantic relationships (Murray 1996). Mothers' beliefs, confidence in their capacity and ability to accomplish and exert control over motivations, behaviours and social environment have been established as a major factor in maternal wellbeing and adaptation (Bandura 1997; Fournier 2002; Stockman and Altmaier 2001). Such positive views may facilitate and foster maternal desires in making the decision to become a mother. Although feelings of ambivalence are also present at this stage, similar to the beginning of romantic relationships, they will be placated with the high expectations of idyllic maternal desires and future expectations.

What happens when optimistic expectations are not matched by later experiences? Studies have shown that women with a high sense of self-efficacy seem better able to cope with challenges in early motherhood (Harwood *et al.* 2007; Teti and Gelfand 1991). The relationship between this self-efficacy and spirituality is supported by the research of Professor Albert Bandura.[3] According to his empirically well-supported social learning theory, a key facilitator of most forms of human behaviour is perceived self-efficacy (Bandura 1986).

Self-efficacy perceptions may strongly influence: a person's motivation to persevere in the face of difficulty; a person's tendency to think optimistically versus pessimistically; the ability to manage aversive emotions; and a person's tendency to interpret relevant events as benign rather than emotionally perturbing (Bandura 1997). The experience of mediators and the specific skills that have been found relevant in the practice of self-efficacy are in the domain of spiritual activities and practices. Following Bandura's research, the studies of Doug

Oman (University of Berkeley) and Carl Thoresen (Stanford University) (Oman and Thoresen 2003; 2007) showed that spirituality involves high-level learned skills related to wise living and effective self-regulation.

Oman *et al.* 2012 related the process of spiritual modelling to the way people learned spiritual behaviour, such as compassion, forgiveness and devotion for themselves and others. It is the cultivation of these self-efficacy spiritual-specific skills that assisted the new mothers in the journey from unconscious desires, expectations and ideal maternal scenarios to the wise consciousness where the authentically real nature of maternal reality is encountered. Mothers in this study often credited self-compassion, kindness and forgiveness as mediators in the difficult task of adaptation to the new reality of motherhood:

> Just sadness, and a kind of a grief for ... but compassion for me as well at that time, and coming to understand that given all the circumstances and where I was at, I don't think it could have been any different, you know, so sort of compassion and forgiveness for myself, but acknowledging that I think that experience made me better.
>
> (Sophia's transcript)

> The resources you need are patience, patience is the first one and kindness. Patience and kindness.
>
> (Serena's transcript)

> This is it, yeah, and it's about managing expectations. You know, what did you think this was going to be like, what were you expecting? But you hear it so often, 'Nobody told us'.
>
> (Dana's transcript)

These spiritual mediators are at the core of spiritual intelligence qualities, as described previously in Chapter 5. Both Oman's research and spiritual intelligence theorists' studies show that such spiritual mediators may act as emotional regulators in the face of maternal difficulties. These spiritual mediators are an attempt to search for identity, belongingness, meaning, health or wellness (Oman *et al.* 2012). In the face of paradox and complexity, it is important then for the mother to enter the liminal space of birth with a well-supported external and internal structure. The preparation for birth is paramount for a smooth passing through the transition. Prenatal classes will assist in incorporating spiritual skills/ mediators in facing labour and birth.

Passing through the transition: birth experiences

Many studies exist that regard birth as a spiritual experience (Callister 2010; Moloney 2007; Parratt 2010; Rosato *et al.* 2006). Pregnancy and childbirth may be perceived as spiritual events because of the miraculous processes involved. Birth narratives often provide insights into the connection between childbearing and lived spirituality through significant, rich narrative data (Callister 2004). In Table 6.1: A Literature Survey of Spirituality in the Context of Motherhood (p. 100), nearly three decades of research showed that half of the maternal literature surveyed identified birth as a spiritual experience. The rest of the studies were about the significance and benefits that midwives can bring through assisting the birthing woman in a spiritually conscious manner.

Women's birth experiences in this study were characterised by expectations, trauma, control, shock and perfectionism. All of these subthemes have been elaborated upon by the mothers in trying to understand the 'passing through the threshold of birth', a place where two births always occurred: the birth of the child and the birth of the mother. In this double birth, a new world of inner wisdom dawned.

Spiritual embodied knowing

Undoubtedly, birth is an embodied experience. A recent thesis entitled 'Feeling Like a Genius: Enhancing Women's Changing Embodied Self During First Childbearing' (Parratt 2010), explored the connection between body and spirituality in the birthing mother. The study stated that the mothers conceptualised the self as a holder of 'spiritual knowing' through the experience of 'embodied knowing'. This spiritual knowing is an inner knowing and contains resources that the mother needs to connect to in order to reach her 'intrinsic power'. This process of birthing inner knowing is very complex. The cultural, historical and social image of maternal bodies has fluctuated from idealisation to degradation through the centuries. As long as such dualities are operating, the integration and connectedness needed in the process of taking hold of inner wisdom are hindered.

In the interviews, some insights can be gleaned towards the difficulty in reaching this internal power. Some of the mothers were very disappointed with the birth to the point of blaming themselves because it did not go the way it was expected. Socio/cultural formed parental philosophy and belief systems are very much in operation here. Many mothers in the study were for example keen for a 'natural birth' (without any medical intervention, including pain relief). Such expectations may reveal a form of 'tyranny of perfection'.

What happens once the body 'fails' to deliver, is what one of the mothers grieved about. It is in such situations that the mother needs adequate self-reflection skills to connect with her 'inner knowing'. The spiritual capacity of self-acceptance is crucial in avoiding the self-surveillance and the self-control to which mothers may submit themselves. The experience of a difficult birth can take years to recover from. Other mothers may be truly disappointed with their bodies and their capacity to birth. Self-acceptance, however, denotes a 'let go', and an 'entering into the unknown' of the birth experience without judging either body, mind or spirit.

This study revealed how birth narratives are filled with pain, joy, sadness, disappointment, love, shock, trauma and many other feelings that are even contradictory in themselves. It is similar to the experience described by the Sufi master Rumi in his poem, 'The Guest House':

> The entertainment of all the joy, depression, meanness, awareness, sorrow as each guest may be clearing you out for some new delight. The dark thought, the shame, the malice: meet them at the door laughing and invite them in. Each has been sent as a guide from beyond.
>
> (Rumi 2004, 109)

A spiritual capacity for embodied knowing requires the ability to invite and entertain physical 'suffering' and the ability to 'engage actively with the uncomfortable and comfortable feelings' without 'judging one's self'. Reflective self-acceptance as a spiritual practice has been found to mediate transformation and growth in the transition to motherhood (Akerjordet 2010). This self-acceptance relieves the feelings of 'judging one's self'. Self-acceptance is complicated for women. Such acceptance for women is often seen as distorted, due to the destructive cultural messages that they receive and internalise, and the maladaptive thinking that they subsequently develop. Some mothers in the interviews expressed it this way:

> I started to train as a pregnancy yoga teacher and that part of addressing my own experience of giving birth and to sort of debrief and face into sort of all the emotions I was still holding on to about it. But I suppose it's just that acceptance that that's how life is, you know, to let go and not be in control.
>
> (Sophia's transcript)

> I still today read stories about people who have these amazing births with no drugs at all and I just think, 'I can't understand why it was so different for me and do we all feel pain differently or do I just have a low threshold that I didn't know I had or is it to do with preparation' ... I suppose what I'm more saying is acceptance.
>
> (Ann's transcript)

Post-transition: postnatal experiences

Most of the interview data produced narratives about postnatal experiences. There were many themes that mothers felt were important during this period. The themes that were cited most by them in the postnatal experiences were instinctual knowledge, identity, connections, change and transformation.

Instinctual knowledge: maternal bodily and intuitive knowing

Instinctual knowledge was the theme most discussed in the interviews. How the mothers in this study refer to daily decisions of minding a baby (sleeping patterns, attachment, feeding, etc.) and later on of caring for a child (activities, education) was related to the engagement of a maternal instinctual knowledge. The mother is constantly trying to reduce cognitive dissonance (Festinger 1957; Harmon-Jones and Mills 1999). Dissonance is inconsistency between behaviours and professed beliefs. This dissonance can generate physiological and emotional signs of distress. Caring for a new baby puts the mother's trust, safety and knowledge into question from the very beginning.

Postmodern motherhood is a challenging act, as self-criticism, guilt and perfection seem to be operating in mothers' psyches as never before. The role of spirituality in combating these negative feelings attached to motherhood may be learning to acknowledge and trust intuitive experiences. It may help mothers to recognise an inner source of truth that enables them to grow spiritually.

In the literature, it has been proposed that humans possess a knowledge instinct; that is, a drive to create realistic internal models of the world. This involves developing mental representations that are as consistent as possible across different hierarchical levels of the brain (Perlovsky 2001; 2006).

Instinctual knowledge involves the individual engaging in the highest levels of the mind hierarchy. It also involves the conscious and the unconscious, the conceptual and the emotional, language and thinking (Harmon-Jones *et al.* 1996).

Mothers often express that they have a unique understanding of their children's needs (maternal knowledge), frequently based on intuition (the gut feeling):

> I was used to being professional and being successful and [a] good decision maker and being in control. I changed my job at a year so I could be home and the job was beside the house and even though the hours were the same in fact I could come home at lunch. So I felt … go with your gut. Yeah I think you would lose a lot by not going with your gut.
>
> (Clare's transcript)

> It's a constant change and it's an evolving thing that it changes to meet the needs of the children at their different ages and stages.
>
> (Serena's transcript)

> You'll only have knowledge by being open with each other and sharing experiences and learning from each other's experiences, you know, and I think the medical profession is still not willing to learn from us, they think they are the experts but we are the experts as well. They should be learning from us.
>
> (Barbara's transcript)

Mothers also spoke of a bodily and instinctual knowledge that they 'engage' in in daily decision-making and also in making meaning of the experience:

People will say, everything really, just put them on the bottle and would you not try a soother and leave them to cry, they are fine for five minutes or anything, oh I wouldn't put those shoes on him all of that stuff you know. It is often what your body or your gut tells you or what you know is not what intellectually what people are telling you so.

(Clare's transcript)

A connection, the body, absolutely, that connection, and also just that relaxing time out away from everybody else. I went into open spaces and opening breastfed, but I never had any embarrassment around it, I knew how to do it without people even knowing, you know? I was good at it, in the end.

(Eve's transcript)

It's working, it's working, you know, your body is doing what your body's meant to do and your baby's doing what your baby's meant to do. It's getting people to actually trust that. It's not all and inconvenience, you know, this is it working at its very best, you know.

(Dana's transcript)

The help is really ... helping them to trust in their own instincts, that they know it's not telling anybody what to do, or saying, 'I'd do it this way'. It's just sort of support, support.

(Sophia's transcript)

These thoughts coincide with studies that have shown that maternal intuition plays a key role in infant feeding practices, with 'gut feelings' being the most powerful determinant for mothers in deciding whether to breast or bottle feed (Heinig *et al.* 2009). Intuition appears to function in situations where mothers are susceptible to blame, and in which the mothers' choices oppose recommendations.

Therefore, there are many spiritual tools or capacities that mothers can employ to fight against the maternal self-policing that commonly overwhelms them during this period and also later on. Mothers in this study underwent a process of becoming more aware of this bodily and instinctual knowledge. Much of the instinctual knowledge is embedded in self-awareness and occurs in everyday living. Intuition as consciousness also functions 'beyond' cognition and thus is interlinked with spirituality. Neurobiologist Damasio clearly showed that it is the sense of our body-selves that we frequently consult when someone asks what we are feeling (Damasio 1999). This instinctual knowledge may be latent consciousness that manifests itself as an 'instinct' before it is fully remembered that something 'feels' right or wrong.

This maternal knowledge (bodily and intuitive) seems to be crucial for the wellbeing of the mother and the baby. Such knowing consists in the construction of personal meaning, and it is a vehicle for understanding and evaluating mothers' helpful meaningful emotions, desires and beliefs for their adjustment to the transition. Transpersonal theorists explain these modes of knowledge (bodily and instinctual) as a dissolution of rational thinking (Hart and Nelson 2000).

Identity: loss, change and discovery

Mothers spoke extensively in the interviews about the loss, change and transformation of their own identity in the transition to motherhood. In spirituality literature, a 'spiritual crisis' reflects a form of identity crisis where drastic changes to the individual's meaning system occurs (Lukoff *et al.* 1995). When this identity crisis happens in the context of motherhood, a meaningful context is needed to integrate the experiences (Bragdon 1993). The struggle to integrate a new maternal identity was evident in some comments:

> There's also sometimes I feel like a loss of identity in a kind of a way, but yet it's not really, I suppose it's just a change in who I am, but I sometimes feel afraid that I'll just, that I'm so submerged in motherhood, that that's all I'm ever going to be.
>
> (Sophia's transcript)

> That joy of motherhood was stripped away from me by them because I hadn't expected that joy of motherhood and they took it away from me for six months in hospital and then I had to work, work, work to regain that ... to give myself identity again.
>
> (Barbara's transcript)

> That's the hard part where you think ... and this whole thing about getting back in to your jeans and getting back out there and everything, that is the piece that is hard. You have to accept, there are other parts of me now, there is a dependency. I think there is a whole drive in to get back in your jeans, get out there, go out with the girls, put them in a crèche, have them sleeping all night, they are grand, they are grand, they are grand. You will get your life back OK but it is all about ignoring your children and ignoring the connection with your children in order to try and maintain that old life. So I think what you really just need is to embrace it [the new life].
>
> (Clare's transcript)

The maternal identity crisis occurs on many different levels: social, psychological, economic and physical. Women occupy a new position in the system of social relations and attain a new social role – that of a mother. A woman's ideas about herself as a mother, and the social expectations of the people around her, will influence the need for a re-structuring of the personal sense of self. Before that re-structuring happens, a disintegration that threatens the women's sense of self is present (Callister 2010; Darvill *et al.* 2010). Most feelings experienced by the mother are very intense in nature and they are in danger of infiltrating all aspects of the mother's everyday living. Some mothers expressed these intense feelings as:

> I find it very hard to trust, you know, and to just be. And it's because I've been there and I've sort of being very insecure, sort of slightly in shock new mother.
>
> (Sophia's transcript)

> I was kind of beating myself up, thinking I was doing something wrong, so … I found my first maternity leave really hard. It was really just the first six months I found really hard. I still feel sad when I look back on it really, because it was just lonely and I think there's a lot of lonely mums out there.
>
> (Ann's transcript)

> I found and I have always found it very hard being at home all day. I find that really hard. I would get depressed you know. The hard thing was going back to work. I had to go back to work when he was four and a half months old. Baby wouldn't look at me, she missed me too much.
>
> (Clare's transcript)

> That transition it was so hard. I felt a disaster. I just felt so stupid by comparison with everybody else. Everybody was functioning.
>
> (Barbara's transcript)

The impact of these feelings and new experiences on the internal framework of the mother is that the ego cannot control them. Has there been much change in the inter-subjectivity of uncertainty or intense vulnerability and lack of control? Transpersonal experiences are those that are characterised by the loss of 'ego boundaries'. The question that arises out of this maternal crisis is: is the transition to motherhood an experience that forces us to go beyond the individual ego? How can mothers use their spiritual innate capacities to alleviate this ongoing process? Experiences that go beyond the ego are intrinsically spiritual experiences.

As discussed in Chapter 3, spirituality may be subjected to the higher states, but also to the 'lower dynamics'. In the humanistic understanding of spirituality, the 'spirit' transcends the 'ego' and the 'psyche'. Spirit may be conscious but also unconscious. The lower dynamics are an important part of the woman's psyche. Transcending the ego is not possible if the mother is not fully conscious and aware of her ego unique processes. Trying to achieve the higher states without knowing the lower dynamics is unrealistic, and even dangerous for the psychospiritual wellbeing of the individual. The psyche is enspirited: the human core of spirituality is the mind as psyche and spirit (Helminiak 1996), therefore, they are intimately connected.

The human spirit grows by getting to know this unconscious part of the spirit and transforming how it affects life. The transpersonal dimension of spirituality is concerned with the awareness or consciousness that is no longer confined exclusively to the individual ego. Current academic dialogue has described how these states are related to self-identity, being and consciousness, in which self-identity becomes integrated into a 'deeper' or 'higher' perspective of the world. Themes such as ambivalence, over-identification, regression, repression, hostility, confusion and separation are seen as being implicit in the maternal crisis (Akerjordet 2010; Barlow 1997; Beck 2002; Liamputtong 2007; Walker 2007).

An example in which the lower dynamics are interrelated with the higher ones can be seen at birth. Self-transcendence is the experience of extending self-boundaries inwardly, outwardly and temporally, to take on broader life perspectives, activities and purposes (Garcia-Romeu 2010). Studies promoting natural birth, without medical intervention, report a spiritual awakening in some mothers (Budin 2001; Peterson 1981). These studies propose that managing or controlling pain in labour will hinder the capacity to challenge the core of one's being. If birth is approached without fear, control and anxiety, the person one was before has, to some degree, ceased to exist – and so has the world in which one used to live (Miller 1992).

Birth as a sacred, transpersonal phenomenon has been extensively researched (Ayers-Gould 2000; Baker 1992; Balin 1988; Callister *et al.* 1999; Hall and Taylor 2004; Lahood 2007; Moloney 2007; Sered 1991). Thus, although birth has the immense potential to be a transcendental experience that can empower and assist the mother in the transition, it can also awaken 'lower dynamics' experiences (trauma, abandonment, loss, sadness, grieving) in the mother, which can seriously 'threaten' her sense of self (Budin 2001; Emmanuel *et al.* 2011; Parratt 2008; Parratt and Fahy 2003; Thompson 1996).

This maternal process is unique to every mother. It is unrealistic to think that every woman can enter a natural birth and have a full transcendent experience, as the consequences of that 'psychic-spiritual opening' are quite serious. The psychospiritual make up of every woman is unique, due to her genetic and environmental influences (experiences in childhood and adulthood). The spiritual dimension is about accepting the uniqueness of her embodied experience. Mothers will make a choice about what kind of birth they want to have, but also what they can manage without compromising their own physical and psychospiritual integrity. In the transition to motherhood, the identity crisis is often responded to with fear, anxiety and control. While the 'lower dynamics of the ego' are doing 'their work' by responding with these compensatory feelings in order to protect the mother's ego, there are other spiritual forces that call for integration. The main spiritual force is the search for the 'authentic self'. The philosophical dimension of spirituality is crucial in how human beings operate in their 'desire for authenticity' (Lonergan 1957). Motherhood is an experience that can foster the search for an authentic truth. The purpose of an identity crisis may be the search for that truth within the self. One of the biggest mediators in the maternal identity crisis is acceptance (of internal and external factors). Fighting the feelings that this transition brings seems intrinsically to feed them and exacerbate them.

Living with the answers and the uncertainty that this identity crisis brings was common in most of the mothers in this study:

> You continuously fall short so therefore you doubt yourself. And I have to say I am a person of taking the line of least resistance.
>
> (Serena's transcript)

> Whatever worry you have, when you've resolved that and another one is waiting just to step into its place, because that's what motherhood is. You will constantly worry about them.
>
> (Dana's transcript)

> We live you know, week by week, month by month, not worrying too far into the future. And that's, who would have ever thought? So you don't know when you have children, and you still don't know what's going to face you in a couple of years' time.
>
> (Eve's transcript)

All of them highlighted these feelings at different periods of their lives. This identity crisis does not seem to be linear. It does not occupy a period in the transition and then it is over. The mothers in this study were at different stages in motherhood: some have babies and very young children, others have teenagers and also grown-up children. They all showed that this negotiation within the self does not stop but it goes through stages. The identity crisis at the beginning of the transition (the first year) is crucial in the sense that it will underlie the foundation on which the mother will work during years to come (Barlow 1997).

Through this process, especially when children are young, the notion of space and time is distorted. Children live in the now. They are not particularly interested in the future and their cognitive abilities are not sufficiently developed to dwell on the past, particularly due to a lack of life experience. The mother engages in the 'now' most of the time. To accept what *is* and to realise that *now* is the only opportunity to create change is a spiritual capacity that helps in the transition. The power of living in the present moment has been researched and is put into practice by meditation (mindfulness) or prayer (centring prayer) (Bourgeault 2004; Tolle 2004). Such practices help the mother receptively enter a contemplative mode of presence in which the sensations of the present moment can reach a consciousness state away from the thinking mind. Living in the now is difficult, but it is in the now that life is happening. The mother encounters the lights and the shadows within herself and the difficult task of dealing with ambivalence on a daily basis.

The identity crisis often arises from maternal ambivalence. Once maternal dualities are confronted, maternal feelings of ambivalence rise to the surface. Society fails to facilitate this type of introspection. In fact, it may even be threatening at a societal level. It is challenging to represent the mother in a non-dual way in the current cultural context. This process also takes time; sometimes it takes years for the mother to come to realise the full meaning of becoming a mother. In this ever-evolving engagement with change, every mother constructs a self-supported network that paves the way to mitigate these challenges with her own identity and the needs of the child.

Trans-temporal themes in the transition to motherhood

Connections and change/transformations are trans-temporal themes because they are manifested at diverse points of the transition. Both are significant and relevant in the prenatal, natal and postnatal temporal points in the transition to motherhood.

Connections

The identity crisis often provokes a relational need in the mother. Connections become crucial in the transition to motherhood. Four different subthemes emerged from this: maternal body connections, support of a maternal network, connection with their own mothers and connections with creativity.

Embodied connections: subjectivity and the lived body

Informed by Merleau-Ponty, our subjectivity resides not in our consciousness alone, but in the lived body (Merleau-Ponty 1962). Motherhood represents a major shift in the modes and limits of the body because of the specific object-related and spatial tasks that motherhood prompts. The comportment, motility and spatiality of the maternal body surely shift radically in its newly furnished world (Baraitser 2009).

Mothers in this study firmly believe that the physical connection with their children (holding, breastfeeding, co-sleeping) decreases the feelings of anxiety and empowers them in their maternal role. These practices were recounted in the interviews of meaning production, and most importantly, the practice of breastfeeding seems to help the mother's self-integrity even after a traumatic birth. Breastfeeding has been described as a gift from mother to child and has a wide range of positive health, social and cultural impacts on infant and mother alike (Cidro *et al.* 2015; Renfrew *et al.* 2005; Thomson *et al.* 2015).

Peer support is reported to be a key method to help build social capital in communities. There are not many studies that describe how this can be achieved through a breastfeeding peer support service. This embodied connection serves the spiritual task of meaning production. Mothers recalled this meaning production through breastfeeding as follows:

> I started to go to a breastfeeding support group, and it was a total life-saver for me. I met other mothers like me who were a bit older, first time mums. I made a bunch of great friends and we started up a great social life together. I suppose a community of mothers who I feel normal with and accepted and

support me in the choices that I make as a mother and who I am as a mother.

(Sophia's transcript)

People just try to do it on their own, and they don't always realise that you're better off to just get out there and go to a mum and baby group, go to a breastfeeding group, join baby massage classes or something, you get to speak to other grown-ups and to share all your problems and, I just didn't know that, I just stayed in the house and it was really hard.

(Ann's transcript)

I was also involved in mother and baby groups and breastfeeding support mornings and I met the people who thought like me. And I thought, 'Oh, I've found these people who are like me. They think like me, they take their babies everywhere, they feel that babies have to be close'.

(Serena's transcript)

When you're vulnerable and tired and wrecked, and because I was that little bit older, I was exhausted like I'd never experienced before, and because I was that bit unwell when I had him, I just thought: I can't give up on the breastfeeding, this is part of me and what I do.

(Dana's transcript)

The connection, well I think the breastfeeding first is a real starting point, because you can't pass your baby over, you can't. So that's the first thing, that physical connection through breastfeeding.

(Eve's transcript)

If you look at the way mammals mind their children, you know you are designed to be close and connected so you know the idea of fighting that close connection. It could be overwhelming for people but I think it comes slowly.

(Clare's transcript)

Mothers thrive on the physical closeness with the infant and they attach it to the meaning of validation in the maternal role. Feelings such as doubt, guilt and blame decrease. Although the expectation of touch differs in motherhood, it seems to continue to have clear psychological and social effects on adults (Traina 2011). These spiritual embodied connections (as mothers called them between them and their children) have the capacity to psychically 'hold' the mother in the transition. These connections are another way to combat the maternal identity crisis.

Connections with the personal and the relational self in maternity

Mothers validate themselves by creating, participating in and gathering in 'similar minded' maternal groups. This means that they engage in their mothering practices with other mothers of a similar parental philosophy. Peer support is considered to be an important means of creating social capital through 'individuals and collectives who care about their own and others' wellbeing'. Positive health and wellbeing outcomes associated with peer support relate to increased access to information, knowledge, competencies and development of meaningful social networks (McKenzie 2006, 25).

Isolation in the transition to motherhood has been proven the 'enemy' for a mother's wellbeing. Lonely individuals are more likely to construe their world (and their behaviour) as potentially threatening or punitive. Inner spiritual understanding of the personal self in relation to the relational self can 'save' the mother from constructing a maternal space that is full of anxiety and stagnation. On the other hand, when human beings are going through crises and challenging times, the evolutionary tendency is inner and relational isolation (Cacioppo *et al.* 2003).

Through peer support and the creation of these groups, mothers increase their social and spiritual capital, which is defined as 'networks together with shared norms, values and understandings that facilitate co-operation within or among groups' (Keeley 2007, 103). Mothers use spiritual capital as an important tool in the transition. Spiritual capital has been described as the spiritual practices, beliefs and networks that have an impact on individuals, communities and societies. These practices must transform and develop the individual into a more authentic self (Malloch 2010). Spiritual capital challenges the maternal silence by connections with the inner part of being and also with others.

Susan Maushart, in her book *The Mask of Motherhood*, writes about the 'fronts' that mothers put out to the world while hiding the reality of their experience (Maushart 1999). She calls this 'the mask of motherhood'. This mask can convey courage, serenity and being all-knowing; yet behind the mask mothers feel angry, frustrated, tired, confused and exhausted. According to Maushart, it is the mask of motherhood that keeps women silent about their true feelings and suspicions concerning what they know. This mask is what minimises the extent of women's work in the world.

Spiritual tools such as attentiveness, self-reflection and self-awareness facilitate the mother in creating these networks in which their real experiences are not silenced. Making meaning of their experiences becomes validated in this environment by mothers connecting experientially with other mums. Making meaning is also a constant task in the transition to motherhood. This spiritual capacity is related to the personal self, the relational self and the collective self. The mother learns to navigate and to enhance these parts of herself in order to create a structure that serves her own and the child's wellbeing in the transition (Brewer and Gardner 1996).

These network connections transform maternal isolation into fruitful practices. Spiritual capital is not only about the individual but extends into communities and societies. Eventually mothers want to engage in making a contribution and changing other mothers in the transition. This is a distinct aspect that relates to experientially going through a spiritual awakening in which, consequently, it is crucial to help others who are going through the same experience. It is the transformative quest for social and cultural transformation that must challenge the dominant discourse in society. The creative side of mothers also seems to be enhanced in the transition, and it is related to the need for universal maternal connection and the need to make a difference.

Connections with the creative energy

John O'Donohue wrote: 'the heart of human identity is the capacity and desire for birthing. To be is to become creative and bring forth the beautiful' (O'Donohue 2004, 142). Creativity is about making space and listening deeply to our lives and the world around us. There is an internal opening and newness during birth that can awake a powerful force to create.

All of these processes contribute in significant ways to the creation of meaning in the mothers' lives. The psychologist Rollo May describes creativity as 'the process of bringing something new into being' (May 1975, 39). Jung also believed that creativity was a force that helps us to access this storehouse of images within ourselves and create a sense of meaning. They are the natural and primary language for the psyche (Welch 1982).

The mothers in the study wanted to create meaning of their experiences, and the work of motherhood became, for some of them, the creative energy:

> It gave me so much passion, it gave me a focus in my life. I was organising the postnatal group and then I was involved with committees, you know 'I'm going to change the world'.
>
> (Barbara's transcript)

> I started to train as a pregnancy yoga teacher: that is part of addressing my own experience of giving birth and to sort of debrief and face into sort of all the emotions I was still holding on to about it. What was a traumatic experience for me, I think, made me stronger and made me a more compassionate and understanding teacher, and I suppose supporter of women who are pregnant and given birth and breastfeeding.
>
> (Sophia's transcript)

> Blogging has been the thing that's made me happiest in the last 40 years. You can write down and there's the dual benefit of the therapy side but also of course then the creative side, the feeling that sense of satisfaction when you put something out there. This is like a whole new interesting world for me. I love it, it's brilliant, I love it.
>
> (Ann's transcript)

> The work of a doula, it's like a piece of armour for mothers, it's like insurance. I could 100 per cent support them.
>
> (Dana's transcript)

Creativity is about seeing beneath the surface of things to the depth dimension of the world; developing a relationship to mystery and giving form in a loving and intentional way to our commitments (Paintner 2007). Creativity has also helped mothers in this study with self-identity and power. This spiritual capacity aids the mothers' own transition and promotes the assistance for others. Creativity moves us beyond ourselves in a similar way to spirituality. It is an intangible human capacity of a transcendent nature. Most of the mothers in this study were opened to the creativity that maternity brought for them. They wanted to enrich their own maternal experiences and those of others, by building maternal networks, running yoga/meditation groups, blogging and writing.

Paolo Knill (1999, 45), one of the founders of expressive arts therapy says: 'the practice of the arts, as disciplined rituals of play in painting, sculpting, acting, dancing, making music, writing, story-telling, is and always was a safe container, a secure vessel to meet existential themes, pathos and mystery'. Creativity may act as a 'spiritual container' in the face of maternal challenges, crisis and changes during the transition. Mothers in this study seemed to search for meaning in their experiences to 'create' resources for other mothers within the transition.

Mothers' connection with their own mothers

It seems important to dwell on the connection of the participants in this study with their own mothers in the transition to motherhood, as they are mentioned quite a lot through their transition to motherhood:

> My mother took such great pleasure in having a grandchild. I liked her and I loved her. I think when it comes to motherhood, my huge regret is not having her to ask questions.
>
> (Dana's transcript)

> You quite often see mums with their babies in their buggies and with their own mother. Like it's very, very common. There's a lot of grandmothers looking after babies and helping mums look after babies. So, I think I always felt a bit sad about that that I didn't have my own mum.
>
> (Ann's transcript)

> My mum was a very social person and she passed away when I was 10, and then I got a lovely step-mum four years later; she has been my mother ever since. So she was my mother when I had all my children, and she was very encouraging. I've had a very good experience of strong female family. My grannies on both sides, my aunties who looked after me after my mother

passed away, my aunties that I'm still in close touch with are very strong women.

(Serena's transcript)

My mother was fantastic, she was great, she was wonderful with the babies. And never told me what to do because she knew I was learning.

(Eve's transcript)

My mother, the day after my wedding, went into a psychiatric hospital. She wasn't there for me so I really missed her, you know, as the youngest child because all the rest of the family emigrated.

(Barbara's transcript)

Their own connections with their mothers seem to be awakening psychospiritual understandings of this process and of themselves. Kristeva poses the question: 'What does a mother want? The answer she provides is that she wants her own mother, even in the figure of the child' (Kristeva 1987, 41). She maintains that it is first and foremost the mother's mother who is encountered in the mother's relationship with the child (Kristeva 1975, 303). The mother's mother is represented as a symbolic container that is present in birth without physically being present. The mother's discourse with her own mother is encountered in the transition to motherhood. It is an archetypal and symbolic discourse even if the mother is not alive. Chernin's ground breaking book: *The Woman Who Gave Birth to Her Mother: Tales of Change in Women's Lives* (Chernin 1999) described this process as a symbolic of self-creation that opens the door to autonomy and achievement; it is a model for breaking the pattern of the endless cycles of blame and forgiveness of mothers within which many women live out their lives. The need for the mother seems to be ambivalent in some cases, and it has been reported that our 'ambivalence metaphor in the self' that mothers keep of her own infantile experiences, are towards their own ambivalence with her own mother (Parker 2005, 19). Being able to reflect onto those symbols, archetypes and metaphors within the self is part of unconscious inner work. Archetypes, symbols and myths are intrinsically related to humans' spiritual quest. Archetypes and symbols within ourselves 'reflect our own struggle to become conscious' (Earl 2001, 282). Our conscious states are 'enforced through the symbols we encounter each day' (Berry 1999, 168). The needs for mothering and to be mothered become a struggle in the maternal transition. Pregnancy, childbirth and the care for the child can 'heavily bear the imprint of the mother' (Balsam 2000, 483).

The awakening of the archetypes and symbols in spirituality is a fertile soil for 'becoming conscious'. Mothers in their own transition to motherhood have experiences of their own internalised mother. To enter these internalised spiritual maternal symbols and archetypes helps new mothers with the duality that women have internalised. Christine Downing, in her book *The Long Journey Home: Re-Visioning the Myth of Demeter and Persephone for Our Time* interprets the visions of Demeter as the all-powerful, all-loving but also devouring, narcissistic mother and cruel and vengeful goddess. All of these facets, albeit that some of them are contradictory in nature, can describe Demeter. Most importantly, she is powerful in all those meanings that define her. In the myth, she 'fights back with rage and violence' and Zeus has to 'give in'[4] (Downing 1994, 116).

Spiritually, for the mother to enter her 'underworld' in relation to her own mother means, again, that she needs to go beyond the dualities that describe what a mother is, or ought to be, according to her own childhood experiences and perceptions. This is a spiritual process because the egoic forces within the mother are negotiated and let go. Narcissistic rages and wounds are exposed in the transition to motherhood, as there is a constant negotiation between dependence needs within the mother and the infant. Those dependence needs are intrinsically related to childhood. The main spiritual capacities that may soothe this process are: compassion, kindness and, most importantly, forgiveness.

Change and transformation

Mothers in this study had diverse emotions, beliefs, insights and values when they were reflecting on their own transition. Their narratives showed that any crisis or challenges that they had encountered have been a fertile soil that assisted their own growth. They reflected on the conscious and the unconscious thoughts and the 'surprises' they met about 'bits' of their personalities that they did not know existed. In order to make meaning of the subjective experience of being a mother and its complex interactions, mothers use spiritual capacities that mediate in the change and transformation. These capacities are: spiritual practices (yoga, meditation and mindfulness), knowledge, journaling (blogging), etc.:

> Because being a parent of three, a lot of the time I feel my head spinning I just got on my yoga mat, had an hour yesterday and I felt so amazing afterwards. I suppose, for me, it is just like coming back to my body again. Yeah, going with the flow, so I don't know, for me at times it's letting go.
>
> (Sophia's transcript)

> I talked to myself in my head with such negativity and self-loathing. That is why mindfulness proved to be such an important development in my life a number of years ago. The main skill I learnt was how to live life with joy.
>
> (Barbara's transcript)

> I'm already writing down about last night, so if something annoying or bad happens, you write it down and get it out of your head and onto the page or the screen, so that's a therapy in itself. It's a silver lining at the end of every challenging experience. It's a non-stop topic. It never stops giving, there's always something new to talk about.
>
> (Ann's transcript)

Spiritual practices: yoga, mindfulness and meditation

These spiritual practices are used by mothers to modify maladaptive thoughts. Anxiety is extinguished during meditation, because the relaxation state replaces the negative reinforcement. Mindfulness meditation helps us to detach and come to full acceptance of thoughts (Hayes 2004). This acceptance through meditation is crucial in the transition to motherhood. All the challenging thoughts, feelings and sensations experienced in the transition can be detached by mothers coming to full acceptance without judging. These spiritual practices foster self-awareness, self-consciousness, self-compassion and constant transformation. The transformation happens at every level: physical, cognitive, emotional and, ultimately, it becomes a spiritual change. The association between meditation, mindfulness and spirituality has been researched with results which sometimes indicate a new expansion in an individuals' inward introspection (Wasner *et al.* 2005), an understanding of a larger humanity and self-compassion (Kristeller and Johnson 2005).

Transformative knowledge and spirituality

Mothers in this study pointed at acquiring knowledge as an intersection in the maternal transformation. This is the era of knowledge as it is readily accessible to everyone. Mothers admitted that new knowledge is powerful in changing how they saw motherhood and how to 'be' within the experience:

> Knowledge is power: I need to know what's ahead of me, and then I'll be able to handle it.
>
> (Dana's transcript)

> Women tend to be so disconnected from their innate wisdom, their sort of innate wisdom and knowledge that's within them and they just, they can't … they find it very hard to trust, you know, and to just be. And it's because I've been there and I've sort of come through that and seen my own journey and being very insecure, sort of slightly in shock new mother, I suppose, I've kind of come full circle to being a mum who now helps other mums and it's just so rewarding.
>
> (Sophia's transcript)

> You see it is not but if you try and do it intellectually you don't get the answer because you are ignoring too much information. Trusting your own self, yeah trust yourself to learn it.
>
> (Clare's transcript)

This findings show that a transformative learning happened in the lives of the mothers. How these changes are manifested affect spirituality. Transformative learning has spiritual aspects to it (Campbell 2010). This maternal knowledge that mothers trust has two different qualities: internal and external. Mothers have the capacity to develop a greater sense of self and meaning through their lived experience. Maternal connection is interrelated with this knowledge, as it takes the mother out of her previous frames of reference and encourages integration with a deeper reality. Maternal support networks are about sharing knowledge and learning from the universality of mothers' experiences. Trust, openness and flexibility are necessary qualities to be available for appropriating this type of knowledge. The emotions that this type of knowledge generate arise spontaneously, beyond the ego's control, therefore, they foster an awareness of the present reality.

Motherhood is an intense experience, but it can become isolated in terms of experiential learning. These findings show that emotions such as fear, doubt, shame, anger and self-mistrust, so often experienced in the transition to motherhood, can be combatted with a transformative knowledge which the mother acquires by means of books, groups or other types of media. This knowledge is spiritually transformative because not only does it take the mother out of her spiritual-psychic isolation, but it also it becomes transpersonal in nature. It is a knowledge that evokes and awakens within the mother aspects of the self previously unknown, unrecognised or unaccepted. The core of the spiritual transformation is about the response that the mother has once those aspects are shown to her clearly. Again, acceptance must be in operation in this spiritual internal change.

These aspects that were often related by the mothers in the interviews need to be fully accepted into the new life in order to make the profound change:

> How it changes you, you know that you have to kind of just abandon it, you know, you know the proper transition is when you stop trying to be the person that you used to be and you just accept the fact I am a mother now and then it is easy.
>
> (Clare's transcript)

> You know, it's a new, it's a whole new job, it's a whole new experience, it's a career change and it's a juggling act and not everybody is perfect, nobody is perfect, you know, it's difficult, it's difficult at times.
>
> (Dana's transcript)

> My focus changed and I think that is something that happens to people when they have children. Priorities change.
>
> (Eve's transcript)

In this process, at the postnatal stage, it is about learning to live with two selves: the old one that it is changing and the new one that is slowly coming into being. Accepting qualities or aspects of the self that are not yet fully developed or even recognised within the mother, is a courageous act. The transition to motherhood shows that unity or wholeness with these new aspects of the self will create a way of living in unity. This concept is intimately related to the 'desire for authenticity', which is the search for knowledge that transforms, accepts and embraces the new realisations of one's life (dark emotions, difficult experiences, joy, ecstasy of love, creative experience). Maternal narratives are part of that vast array of transformative knowledge which connects the mother with all the earlier maternal stories.

Transformational skills

In this study, mothers highlighted a cognizance of their self-knowledge in their awareness of their beliefs, values, attitudes and emotions. There was a conscious awareness and acknowledgement of the skills that are needed in the transition to motherhood. Skills that are mentioned are: selflessness, inquisitiveness, openness, encouragement without criticism, playfulness, patience, acceptance, kindness, patience and good humour. These skills or qualities were seen as crucial in meditating the transformation in the transition. The letting go is part of transcending the egoic self and accepting the changes that are happening on a daily basis in the transition. Acceptance is a major mediator in the transition. In a way, the healing and transformation start happening once the mother has accepted that her 'old self' has disappeared and there is an embracing of the 'new self'. The conundrum was accepting the 'new self', even when it is in progress, even when it seems it is failing, even when it cannot be sensed, even when it is still in 'darkness'.

Conclusions

The constancy of making meaning of the experience seemed to be ongoing. It is a process to evolve into a different kind of being. It is unique for everyone. Spirituality acknowledges that uniqueness is in every individual. Resisting talking and relating in dualities to motherhood, means that every emotion, insight and feeling, no matter how awful or painful they may be, are found to make sense in its context. The skills that mothers kept referring back to in their narrative were: kindness, forgiveness, patience, compassion and openness. These are crucial when there is a 'suffering' and a 'waiting' to become.

As in the heroine's journey, the transition to motherhood is a rite of passage, an awakening to different layers within the self and a leap of faith. If faith is described as the substance of things hoped for, the evidence of things not seen,[5] it is possible to imagine the courage, trust and strength that is needed in the process of the transition to motherhood.

Notes

1 For the full definition, see: www.oxforddictionaries.com/definition/english/illusion.
2 For the full definition, see: www.oxforddictionaries.com/definition/english/expectation?q=expectations.
3 Albert Bandura is a Professor of Psychology at Stanford University. For six decades, he has made contributions to many fields of psychology, including social cognitive

theory, therapy and personality psychology. He is known as the originator of social learning theory and the theoretical construct of self-efficacy.

4 In Ancient Greek mythology, Zeus is the god of sky and thunder and the ruler of the Olympians and Mount Olympus.

5 Hebrews 11:1 (King James Bible).

References

Akerjordet, K. 2010. 'Being in Charge – New Mothers' Perceptions of Reflective Leadership and Motherhood'. *Journal of Nursing Management* 18(4):409–417.

Ayers-Gould, J. 2000. 'Spirituality in Birth: Creating Sacred Space within the Medical Model'. *International Journal of Childbirth Education* 15(1):14–17.

Baker, J. 1992. 'The Shamanic Dimensions of Childbirth'. *Pre- and Peri-natal Psychology Journal* 7(1):5–20.

Balin, J. 1988. 'The Sacred Dimensions of Pregnancy and Birth'. *Qualitative Sociology* 11(4):275–301.

Balsam, R. 2000. 'The Mother within the Mother'. *Psychoanalytic Quarterly* 69(3):465–491.

Bandura, A. 1986. *Social Foundations of Thought and Action: A Social Cognitive Approach*. Englewood Cliffs, USA: Prentice-Hall.

Bandura, A. 1997. *Self-Efficacy – The Exercise of Control*. New York: W.H. Freeman and Company.

Baraitser, L. 2009. *Maternal Encounters. The Ethics of Interruption. Women and Psychology*. London: Routledge.

Barlow, C. 1997. 'Mothering as a Psychological Experience: A Grounded Theory Exploration'. *Canadian Journal of Counselling* 31(3):232–237.

Battersby, C. 1998. *The Phenomenal Woman: Feminist Metaphysics and the Patterns of Identity*. Oxford, UK: Polity Press.

Beck, C. 2002. 'Postpartum Depression: A Metasynthesis'. *Qualitative Health Research* 12(4):453–472.

Benzies, K. 2008. 'Advanced Maternal Age: Are Decisions about the Timing of Child-Bearing a Failure to Understand the Risks?'. *Canadian Medical Association Journal* 178(2):183–184.

Benzies, K., Tough, K., Tofflemire, C., Frick, A., and Faber, C. 2006. 'Factors Influencing Women's Decisions about Timing of Motherhood'. *Journal of Obstetric, Gynecologic, and Neonatal Nursing* 35:625–633.

Berry, T. 1999. *The Great Work: Our Way into the Future*. New York: Three Rivers Press.

Bongaarts, J., and Watkins, S. 1996. 'Social Interactions and Contemporary Fertility Transitions'. *Population and Development Review* 22(4):639–682.

Bourgeault, C. 2004. *Centering Prayer and Inner Awakening*. USA: Cowley Publications.

Bragdon, E. 1993. *Helping People with Spiritual Problems*. Vermont, USA: Lightening Up Press.

Brewer, M., and Gardner, W. 1996. 'Who is this "We"? Levels of Collective Identity and Self Representations'. *Journal of Personality and Social Psychology* 71:83–93.

Budin, W. 2001. 'Birth and Death: Opportunities for Self-Transcendence'. *Journal Perinatal Education* 10(2):38–42.

Cacioppo, J., Hawkley L., and Berntson, G. 2003. 'The Anatomy of Loneliness'. *Current Directions in Psychological Science* 12:71–74.

Callister, L. 2004. 'Making Meaning: Women's Birth Narratives'. *Journal of Obstetric, Gynecologic, and Neonatal Nursing* 3(4):508–518.

Callister, L. 2010. 'Spirituality in Childbearing Women'. *Journal of Perinatal Education* 19(2):16–24.

Callister, L., Semenic, S., and Foster, J. 1999. 'Cultural and Spiritual Meanings of Childbirth: Orthodox Jewish and Mormon Women'. *Journal of Holistic Nursing* 17(3):280–295.

Campbell, K. 2010. *Transformative Learning and Spirituality: A Heuristic Inquiry into the Experience of Spiritual Learning.* PhD Diss., Capella University, Minneapolis, USA.

Chernin, K. 1999. *The Woman Who Gave Birth to Her Mother: Tales of Change in Women's Lives.* San Francisco: Penguin Books.

Cidro, J., Lynelle Z., Herenia P., Lawrence, S., Folster, M., and McGregor, K. 2015. 'Breast Feeding Practices as Cultural Interventions for Early Childhood Caries in Cree Communities'. *BMC Oral Health* 15:49.

Damasio, A. 1999. *The Feeling of What Happens: Body and Emotion in the Making of Consciousness.* New York: Harcourt Brace.

Darvill, R., Skirton, H., and Farrand, P. 2010. 'Psychological Factors that Impact on Women's Experiences of First-Time Mothers: A Qualitative Study of the Transition'. *Midwifery* 26:357–366.

Downing, C. 1994. *The Long Journey Home. Revisioning the Myth of Demeter and Persephone for Our Time.* Boulder, USA: Shambhala Publications.

Earl, M. 2001. 'Shadow and Spirituality'. *International Journal of Children's Spirituality* 6(3):277–288.

Emmanuel, E., Creedy, D., St John, W., and Brown, C. 2011. 'Maternal Role Development: The Impact of Maternal Distress and Social Support following Childbirth'. *Midwifery* 27(2):265–272.

Esbjorn, V. 2003. *Spirited Flesh: An Intuitive Inquiry Exploring the Body in Contemporary Female Mystics.* PhD Diss., Institute of Transpersonal Psychology, Palo Alto, USA.

Festinger, L. 1957. *A Theory of Cognitive Dissonance.* Stanford, USA: Stanford University Press.

Fournier, V. 2002. 'Fleshing out Gender: Crafting Gender Identity on Women's Bodies'. *Body & Society* 8(2):55–77.

Garcia-Romeu, A. 2010. 'Self-Transcendence as a Measurable Transpersonal Construct'. *Journal of Transpersonal Psychology* 42(1):26–47.

Hall, J., and Taylor, M. 2004. 'Birth and Spirituality'. In *Normal Childbirth: Evidence and Debate*, edited by S. Downes, 41–56. Edinburgh, UK: Churchill Livingston.

Harmon-Jones, E., and Mills, J. 1999. *Cognitive Dissonance: Progress on a Pivotal Theory in Social Psychology.* Washington, DC: American Psychological Association.

Harmon-Jones, E., Brehm, J., Greenberg, J., Simon, L., and Nelson, D. 1996. 'Evidence that the Production of Aversive Consequences is Not Necessary to Create Cognitive Dissonance'. *Journal of Personality and Social Psychology* 70:5–16.

Hart, T., and Nelson, P. 2000. *Transpersonal Knowing: Exploring the Horizon of Consciousness.* SUNY Series, Transpersonal & Humanistic Psychology. Albany, USA: State University of New York Press.

Harwood, K., McLean, N., and Durkin, K. 2007. 'First-Time Mothers' Expectations of Parenthood: What Happens When Optimistic Expectations are Not Matched by Later Experiences?'. *Developmental Psychology* 43:1–12.

Hayes, C. 2004. *Mindfulness and Acceptance. Expanding the Cognitive-Behavioural Tradition.* New York: The Guilford Press.

Heinig, M., Ishii, K., Banuelos, J., Campbell, E., O'Loughlin, C., and Vera-Becerra, L. 2009. 'Sources and Acceptance of Infant-Feeding Advice among Low-Income Women'. *Journal of Human Lactation* 25:163–172.

Helminiak, D. 1996. *The Human Core of Spirituality: Mind as Psyche and Spirit.* New York: State University of New York Press.

Hrdy, S. 1999. *Mother Nature: A History of Mothers, Infants, and Natural Selection.* New York: Pantheon Books.

Kach, J., and McGhee, P. 1982. 'Adjustment to Early Parenthood: The Role of Accuracy of Preparenthood Expectations'. *Journal of Family Issues* 3:361–374.

Kaskisaari, M. 1999. 'Taidehalu – Ruumiilliset Kokemukset ja Arjen Järjestys Naisten Taideomaelämäkerroissa' (Desire for Art – Embodied Experiences and the Ordering of Everydayness in Women's Autobiographies). *Naistutkimus-Kvinnoforskning* 12(3):2–17.

Keeley, B. 2007. *Human Capital: How What You Know Shapes Your Life.* Paris: OECD.

Knill, P. 1999. 'Soul Nourishment or the Intermodal Language of the Imagination'. In *Foundations of Expressive Arts Therapy*, edited by S. Levine, and E. Levine, 38–45. Philadelphia, USA: Jessica Kingsley Publications.

Kohler, H. 2001. *Fertility and Social Interaction: An Economic Perspective.* Oxford, UK: Oxford University Press.

Kristeller, J., and Johnson, T. 2005. 'Cultivating Loving Kindness: A Two-Stage Model of the Effects of Meditation on Empathy, Compassion, and Altruism'. *Journal of Religion and Science* 40(2):391–408.

Kristeva, J. 1975. *Desire in Language: A Semiotic Approach to Literature and Art.* New York: Columbia University Press.

Kristeva, J. 1987. *The Kristeva Reader*, edited by T. Moi. New York: Columbia University Press.

Lahood, G. 2007. 'Rumour of Angels and Heavenly Midwives: Anthropology of Transpersonal Events and Childbirth'. *Women and Birth* 20(7):3–10.

Liamputtong, P. 2007. 'When Giving Life Starts to Take the Life out of You: Women's Experiences of Depression after Childbirth'. *Midwifery* 23:77–91.

Liesen, L. 2001. 'Review: Mother Nature: A History of Mothers, Infants, and Natural Selection'. *Politics and the Life Sciences* 20(2):246–248.

Lonergan, B. 1957. *Insight: A Study of Human Understanding.* Toronto: University of Toronto Press.

Lukoff, D., Lu, F., and Turner, R. 1995. 'Cultural Considerations in the Assessment and Treatment of Religious and Spiritual Problems'. *The Psychiatric Clinics of North America* 18(3):467–485.

Malloch, T. 2010. 'Spiritual Capital and Practical Wisdom'. *Journal of Management Development* 29(7/8):755–759.

Maushart, S. 1999. *The Mask of Motherhood: How Becoming a Mother Changes Our Lives and Why We Never Talk about It.* Auckland, New Zealand: Penguin Books.

May, R. 1975. *The Courage to Create.* New York: W.W. Norton & Co.

McKenzie, K. 2006. 'Social Risk, Mental Health and Social Capital'. In *Social Capital and Mental Health*, edited by K. McKenzie, and T. Harpham, 24–38. London: Jessica Kingsley Publishers.

Mercer, R. 2004. 'Becoming a Mother Versus Maternal Role Attainment'. *Journal of Nursing Scholarship* 36:7.

Merleau-Ponty, M. 1962. *The Phenomenology of Perception.* New York: Routledge and Kegan Paul.

Miller, J. 1992. 'The Way of Suffering: A Reasoning of the Heart?'. *Second Opinion* 17(4):21–33.

Moloney, S. 2007. 'Dancing with the Wind: A Methodological Approach to Researching Women's Spirituality around Menstruation and Birth'. *International Journal of Qualitative Methods* 6(1):114–125.

Montgomery, K., Green, T., Maher, B., Tipton, K., O'Bannon, C., Murphy, T., McCurry, T., Shaffer, L., Best, S., and Hatmaker-Flanigan, E. 2010. 'Women's Desire for Pregnancy'. *Journal of Perinatal Education* 19(3):53–61.

Murray, S. 1996. 'The Self-Fulfilling Nature of Positive Illusions in Romantic Relationships: Love Is Not Blind, but Prescient'. *Journal of Personality and Social Psychology* 7(6):1155–1180.

O'Donohue, J. 2004. *Beauty: The Invisible Embrace.* New York: Harper Collins.

Oman, D., and Thoresen, C. 2003. 'Spiritual Modeling: A Key to Spiritual and Religious Growth?'. *The International Journal for the Psychology of Religion* 13:149–165.

Oman, D., and Thoresen, C. 2007. 'How Does One Learn to be Spiritual? The Neglected Role of Spiritual Modeling in Health'. In *Spirit, Science and Health: How the Spiritual Mind Fuels Physical Wellness*, edited by T. G. Plante and C. E. Thoresen, 39–56. Westport, USA: Praeger/Greenwood.

Oman, D., Thoresen, C., Park, C., Shaver, P., Hood, R., and Plante, T. 2012. 'Spiritual Modelling Self-Efficacy'. *Psychology of Religion and Spirituality* 4(4):278–297.

Paintner, V. 2007. 'The Relationship between Spirituality and Artistic Expression: Cultivating the Capacity for Imagining'. *Spirituality in Higher Education Newsletter* 3(2):1–6.

Parker, R. 2005. *The Experience of Maternal Ambivalence. Torn in Two.* London: Virago Press.

Parratt, J. 2008. 'Territories of the Self and Spiritual Practices during Childbirth'. In *Birth Territory and Midwifery Guardianship*, edited by K. Fahy, 39–54. Oxford, UK: Books for Midwives.

Parratt, J. 2010. *Feeling like a Genius: Enhancing Women's Changing Embodied Self during First Childbearing.* PhD Diss., University of Newcastle, Newcastle, Australia.

Parratt, J., and Fahy, K. 2003. 'Trusting Enough to be out of Control: A Pilot Study of Women's Sense of Self during Childbirth'. *Australian Midwifery* 16(1):1522.

Perlovsky, L. 2001. *Neural Networks and Intellect.* New York: Oxford University Press.

Perlovsky, L. 2006. *Toward Physics of the Mind: Concepts, Emotions, Consciousness, and Symbols.* New York: Oxford University Press.

Perrin, D. 2007. *Studying Christian Spirituality.* Oxford, UK: Routledge.

Peterson, G. 1981. *Birthing Normally: A Personal Approach to Childbirth.* Berkeley, USA: Mindbody Press.

Raphael-Leff, J. ed. 2003. *Parent-Infant Psychodynamics: Wild Things, Mirrors and Ghosts.* London: Whurr Publications.

Ravn, M. 2005. 'A Matter of Free Choice? Some Structural and Cultural Influences on the Decision to Have or Not to Have Children in Norway'. In *Barren States: The Population 'Implosion' in Europe*, edited by C. Douglass, 29–48. Oxford, UK: Berg Press.

Renfrew, M., Dyson, L., Wallace, D'Souza, L., McCormick, F., and Spiby, H. 2005. *The Effectiveness of Public Health Interventions to Promote the Duration of Breastfeeding Systematic Review.* London: NICE.

Romo, L., Berenson, A., and Segars, A. 2004. 'Sociocultural and Religious Influences on the Normative Contraceptive Practices of Latino Women in the United States'. *Contraception [Electronic Version]* 69:219–225.

Rosato, M., Mwansambo, C., Kazembe, P., Phiri, T., Sokso, S., Lewycka, S., Kunyenge, B., Vergnano, S., Osrin, D., Newell, L., and Costello, M. 2006. 'Women's Groups Perceptions of Maternal Health Issues in Rural Malawi'. *Lancet* 368:1180–1188.

Rumi, J. 2004. *The Essential Rumi. New Expanded Edition.* New York: HarperOne Press.

Sered, S.1991. 'Childbirth as a Religious Experience? Voices From an Israeli Hospital'. *Journal of Feminist Studies in Religion* 7(2):7–18.

Sevon, E. 2005. 'Timing Motherhood: Experiencing and Narrating the Choice to Become a Mother'. *Feminism Psychology* 15(4):461–482.

Stockman, A. F., and Altmaier, E. 2001. 'Relation of Self-Efficacy to Reported Pain and Pain Medication Usage during Labour'. *Journal of Clinical Psychology in Medical Settings* 8(3):161–166.

Teti, D., and Gelfand, D. 1991. 'Behavioural Competence among Mothers of Infants in the First Year: The Mediational Role of Self-Efficacy'. *Child Development* 65:918–929.

Thompson, S. 1996. 'Barriers to Maintaining a Sense of Meaning and Control in the Face of Loss'. *Journal of Personal and Intrapersonal Loss* 1:333–357.

Thomson, G., Balaam, M., and Hymers, K. 2015. 'Building Social Capital through Breastfeeding Peer Support: Insights from an Evaluation of a Voluntary Breastfeeding Peer Support Service in North-West England'. *International Breastfeeding Journal* 10:1–15.

Tolle, E. 2004. *The Power of Now: A Guide to Spiritual Enlightenment.* Vancouver, Canada: Namaste Publishing.

Traina, L. 2011. *Erotic Attunement. Parenthood and the Ethics of Sensuality Between Unequal.* Chicago, USA: University of Chicago Press.

Walker, R. 2007. *Baby Love: Choosing Motherhood after a Lifetime of Ambivalence.* New York: Riverhead Books.

Wasner, M., Longaker, C., Fegg, M. J., and Borasio, G. 2005. 'Effects of Spiritual Care Training for Palliative Care Professionals'. *Palliative Medicine* 19:99–104.

Welch, J. 1982. *Spiritual Pilgrims: Carl Jung and Theresa of Avila.* New York: Paulist Press.

Wylie, M. 1979. 'The Effect of Expectations on the Transition to Parenthood'. *Sociological Focus* 12:323–329.

9 Implications for the future

There are studies on spirituality research that come close to new frontiers within spiritual care in diverse maternal health contexts. Maternal crisis has been researched in the context of the spirituality of mothers who have high-risk pregnancies, stillborn deliveries and miscarriages (Mann *et al*. 2007; 2008, Nuzum *et al*. 2014; 2015). These studies highlighted the necessity of spiritual care training for people who care for mothers. Studies show that chaplains involved in perinatal healthcare ministry lack spiritual-care training in dealing with traumatic events in childbirth (Nuzum *et al*. 2014; 2015). Nuzum *et al*. (2015) recommended that carers who are in the perinatal healthcare ministry need to engage in structured theological reflection and reflective practices.

Other studies have highlighted the difficult decisions around cancer treatments that some mothers need to make in order to preserve the life of their baby. They indicate that mothers relied on their spirituality for the management of stress and hardship related to the cancer and the new baby (Manning and Radina 2015; Snodgrass 2012). There are many studies which have proved that spirituality is beneficial in times of crisis and trauma, either in mental health and addictions contexts. Individuals recovering from addictions, trauma or crisis frequently cite spirituality as a helpful influence. However, there is little research about whether or how spirituality could be incorporated into formal treatment in a manner that is sensitive to individual differences.

A study used focus groups in the treatment of substance abuse and found that nearly all participants agreed that integrating a spiritual discussion into formal treatment is preferable to current methods (Heinz *et al*. 2010). In maternal contexts, Crowther and Hall (2015) believe that spirituality still remains on the periphery of current discourse about childbirth, and that most of the spiritual care guidelines are insufficient for assessing the unique lived-experience of childbirth. The researchers felt that the unique spiritual experiences are lost in a culture of ticking boxes.

Spiritual support and education have also been highlighted as a need for the caregivers as they are ones who facilitate mothers. Recent studies show the importance of spiritual assessment and spiritual support for caregivers, who exhibit spiritual pain and psychological distress while caring for patients with advanced cancer. In the same manner, recent studies on secondary spiritual crisis experienced by maternal caregivers have described compassion and empathy fatigue, post-traumatic stress disorder and secondary traumatic stress as potential consequences of caring for women who experience birth trauma or perinatal bereavement (Davies and Coldridge 2015; Leinweber and Rowe 2010; Rice and Warland 2013). Also, in chaplaincy, research showed that the deep and profound spiritual crisis within mothers can cause secondary spiritual crisis within the chaplains in their own beliefs, values and personal faith (Nuzum *et al.* 2015).

Through this study, I argue that spirituality is common to all mothers regardless of their beliefs and value systems. Spirituality in this framework is understood anthropologically and is embedded in social, cultural, historical, linguistic and biological realities. This framework encompasses the understanding of spirituality as a quest for meaning, as well as a search for the true self. It is a journey of consciousness, and for some people is a reconnection with a 'Higher Consciousness'.

The maternal spiritual process is unique for every mother in what she wants to search for within herself, and/or beyond herself. The aim of this study was ultimately to create a maternal-spiritual framework so as to design an appropriate spirituality model that is capable of facilitating and empowering the maternal learning of important spiritual skills. The important questions in creating this maternal-spiritual framework are: how does spirituality assist a woman through the maternal transition? What are the spiritual tools/capacities that mothers employed? Do spiritual capacities help in the transition to motherhood, and how are they used by the mother? What were the spiritual changes for the woman once she had become a mother?

Up to now, most studies have researched spirituality and motherhood with a focus on the liminal space of the transition (birth). Some studies have also researched the role of midwives and how they can assist the new mother spiritually. Overall, the literature revealed a lack of research in this area regarding: (a) how the mother can use spiritual skills; and (b) understanding spirituality as being at the core of the major maternal life transition.

I have employed four building blocks from the literature of spirituality to elucidate an exploratory framework for the study of maternal spirituality: transpersonal psychology, humanistic psychology, spiritual intelligence and the theory of spiritual crisis. For purposes of analysis, the transition was divided into three time points: pre-transition (prenatal experiences), passing through the transition (birth) and post-transition (postnatal experiences). Six main themes located in the temporal points of pre-transition and post-transition illustrate the diverse spiritual needs of the mother at each stage. These needs remain sensitive to the themes and trends that emerged in the interviews data. These themes and their relationship with current research are summarised below.

Key findings

The desire/expectations and illusions concerning mothering emerged as a central theme in prenatal experiences. All mothers in this study constructed personal life meaning around reproduction and the personal fulfilment that being a mother would provide. Although there has been some research around the desire for reproduction, there is little or none about the spiritual meaning that mothers attached to this desire in their own lives. The non-desire for reproduction and voluntary childlessness is still controversial in a culture that reveres motherhood as central to feminine identity. The spiritual meanings that women attach to their lives when they consciously choose not to have children are also under-researched.

Spiritually embodied knowing was the theme that emerged during the passing through of the transition (birth). Birthing, inner knowing and inner wisdom were spiritual maternal resources at the core of an experience of empowerment in mothers giving birth. This key finding is very significant in a culture that is ambivalent of women's bodies. The inter-relation between women's bodies and spirituality in birth is an exciting line of inquiry. Birthing as spiritual transformation has scarcely been investigated.

Instinctual knowledge was a postnatal theme that mothers employed from their everyday maternal experiences. The maternal instinctual knowledge protects and secures the integrity and wellbeing of mother and baby. The transformative instinctual knowledge that mothers employ during their transition impacts on the overall wellbeing of mothers and babies. Very little is known about that internal knowledge. In contemporary society, the market place thrives on maternal books, videos, courses and all type of experts advising mothers how to mother. Studies are needed on how mothers can access their internal knowledge and what skills are needed in order to do it.

Identity crisis was the theme that ran through all three points of the transition. The drastic, crucial and intense feelings experienced in the transition impacted greatly on the mothers' meaning systems. Identity crisis is often researched in pathological psychological conditions. More research on how this identity crisis impacts on non-pathological events is needed. The transition to motherhood does not need to be pathologised. It needs to be investigated from a spiritual holistic view to assist the mother with all the difficult feelings, behaviours and new social/cultural and economic challenges that that may bring.

The experience of being connected was a trans-temporal theme that helped mothers to negotiate their social capital, subjective experiences, creativity and their relationship with themselves and others. The term 'being connected' appeared in spirituality studies as a spiritual health indicator (Hitchcock *et al.* 2003; Hover-Kramer 2002). The sense of 'being connected' is deeply personal (connectedness with one's inner self) and inter-relational (being in a meaningful relationship with others). Studies on the meaning and definition of spiritual maternal connections may decode the intricacies of how mothers connect with themselves after the birth. The type of connections that mothers need to adjust well to their new role is paramount in understanding spiritual connections as a maternal health indicator.

Change and transformation was also a trans-temporal theme which emerged in the emphasis on the importance of spiritual practices, new knowledge (transformative learning) and new skills in the transition to motherhood. Although this study has outlined some, more research is needed on the significance of spiritual practices that can transform mothers' challenging experiences and also on the spiritual capacities that may be transformative if applied in the transition to motherhood.

Implications for future research

New research on maternal studies in the discipline of spirituality would benefit from engaging in an integral approach in which science, religion, philosophy, transpersonal studies and humanistic psychology integrate the physical, emotional, mental and spiritual aspects of the motherhood experience across the three key temporal stages identified in this study. Integral studies bring and link together concepts, practices and theories from a wide range of academic disciplines to try to create a 'meta-vision' of any particular subject of study. Integral studies are examples of a new level of consciousness in human development (Wilber 1986; 1997; 2007).

The main theorists in the area of integral studies are: transpersonal writer, Ken Wilber (Wilber 2007), cultural philosopher, Jean Gebser (Gebser 1986), Professor of Psychology, Clare Graves (Graves 1970), social psychologist, Don Beck (Beck and Cowan 2005) and integral theorist, Mark Woodhouse (Woodhouse 1996).[1] Integral studies are sophisticated, timely and contemporary manifestations of the general perception of the global spiritual transformation.

In particular, seven core areas that this study introduced could be further expanded in future research:

1   *Maternal anxiety/depression.* These areas have been extensively researched in the literature from a psychological and biological framework. However, the 'new' maternal anxiety which is socially constructed today needs to be further researched within a non-pathological framework. The relationship between spirituality and the anxiety-laden demands of being a mother in the twenty-first century provides a fertile soil for understanding how the inner core of motherhood has evolved from previous generations. The challenges of the new anxiety and the spiritual practice interventions that may be helpful in combatting it are exciting new lines of investigation in spirituality research.

2   *Birth experiences.* These have been researched in many transpersonal studies (Ayers-Gould 2000; Baker 1992; Balin 1988; Budin 2001; Burns 2015; Callister 2010; Crowther 2013; Fisher and Bickel 2005; Klassen 2005; Lahood 2007; Sempruch 2005; Sered 1991). However, most of these transpersonal studies need to be expanded beyond the date of the birth and the later points in the timeline of maternal transition. Transpersonal experiences which introduce an individual to the space beyond the ego have crucial consequences in the life of an individual. To comprehend how such experiences at the time of a birth have an impact in the postnatal period can

help to conceptualise how the mother's self-understanding may be transformed and expanded later on in the transition to motherhood.

3 *Spiritual intelligence capacities.* Personal meaning production, conscious awareness, self-reflection/reflexivity, creativity and transpersonal orientation need to be further investigated in each of the three temporal phases of the transition to motherhood. A better understanding of these capacities could form part of transformative learning for the mothers in education, health and psychological settings, if they were incorporated into maternal courses.

4 *Maternal connections.* Current research on how human connections are changing in the twenty-first century is an exciting field of enquiry. The virtual social connections (Twitter, Facebook, blogging, Instagram, forums, etc.) are assisting mothers in creating/having a voice that would have been unthinkable in the past. An investigation into the relationship within the 'new connections' (the virtual maternal agora) and their implicit spiritual explorations could show how the subjective mothering experiences impacts on the spiritual evolution of a large number of mothers in the world simultaneously.

5 *Maternal consciousness.* Neurobiologically, transpersonal experiences in the transition to motherhood could be further researched in order to elucidate the mechanisms used by the mother to access them. Transpersonal experiences not only offer access to the dynamics of psychospiritual change and transformation, but also have the capacity to provide a scientific understanding of the processes and states of the mind (perception, emotion, memory and thinking) in such an altered phase. Studies relating to phenomena such as maternal precognition experiences, perceptions, dreams or other psi experiences (such as apparitions, visions, out-of-body experiences, near-death experiences) would be very beneficial in elucidating the neurophysiological dimensions of consciousness in the transition to motherhood.

6 *Maternal ambivalence.* Many psychological studies have investigated maternal ambivalence, but there is a need to expand the research so as to include the impact of maternal ambivalence on the spirituality of the mother. The spiritual practices and capacities which may be employed by mothers to dialogue with such ambivalence require specific attention in order to discover what, for the mother, may lead to reconciliation of the dichotomies that she is compelled to enter, from the very beginning of the transition.

7 *Maternal/spiritual embodiment.* More research needs to be undertaken in the domains of adoptive, fostering and surrogate mothering, while acknowledging that surrogacy is somewhat different since although the baby is frequently raised by the biological mother, the foetus was implanted, nourished and born from another woman. Further investigation regarding the impact of spirituality on mothers in other new scenarios of assisted reproduction will elucidate the relationship of motherhood with spirituality when motherhood has not been an 'embodied experience' during pregnancy and birth.

Implications for future practice by professionals

Many professionals who are involved in the area of maternal health and education could benefit from the findings of this study of themes and trends in spirituality during the transition to motherhood.

Maternal educators (hospital, college, university) could foster a spiritually-grounded transformative maternal education that could facilitate the mother during the prenatal, birth and postnatal transition. Holistic maternal education studies are still in their infancy, but they are extremely important for the well-supported external and internal structures that mothers require for empowerment in the face of a profound life-altering event. Ante- and postnatal classes would benefit by incorporating a framework of spiritual transformation into their programmes in a manner akin to the way stress management education was transformed by the introduction of mindfulness-based stress reduction.

Maternity health staff who assist the mother (midwives, students, lactation consultants, nurses, chaplains, doctors) could also benefit from courses that are holistic in nature and do not standardise the 'experiences' of mothers. A recent study has recommended an increased embeddedness, into midwifery practice, of empathic understanding, appreciation of the notion of 'birth as sacred' and the practice of spiritual care (Moloney and Gair 2015). Natural birth, breastfeeding or other maternity practices cannot be standardised for all mothers, as the meaning construction regarding such practices will vary from woman to woman. A transformative spiritually-informed practice in the transition will enhance maternal agency.

Maternity researchers/scholars will also benefit from this study. The exploratory framework (transpersonal psychology, humanistic psychology, philosophical practice, spiritual intelligence and the theory of spiritual crisis) can serve, and be applied to, future maternal spiritual care research in diverse settings. The transformational skills outlined in this study may be researched in various maternal contexts, in order to explore their effectiveness in facilitating the maternal transition.

Chaplains who are often at the front line of maternal caregivers will also benefit from a deeper knowledge of the maternal spiritual capacities singled out by this study in Chapter 6. These capacities not only improve the mother's sense of self and her maternal agency, but they also explicate the spiritual role of caregivers towards the mothers.

Psychological staff (counsellors, psychotherapists, psychiatrists, psychologists) have an important role in the maintenance of the wellbeing of the emotional world of mothers. These professionals will benefit by incorporating psychospiritual dimensions into the therapies they employ. Maternal psychospiritual therapy groups are often highly important in assisting mothers in their transition.

Most professionals will benefit from maternal psychospiritual courses in assisting mothers. Professionals need to acquire spiritual skills in order to facilitate mothers in their transition. Spiritual education is a holistic, growthful, experiential, reflective and transformative process that needs to involve both the maternal educator and the mothers. Maternal courses need to foster all the different processes and ways of knowing, not only the conventional forms of intellectual functioning and critical thinking but also the educational value of unique maternal personal experience, the wisdom of the maternal body and forms of creative expression: such spiritual practices like meditation, poetry, story, arts, journaling, contemplative inquiry and reflective practices. The aim of maternal education is about benefiting the self and others and allowing mothers to find their unique, authentic voice and to cultivate spiritual values and qualities: self-compassion, insight, interconnectedness, intuition, mindfulness and self-empathy.

Maternal educators need to be aware of their own processes of awareness and inner change as they guide mothers. This is a journey of self-discovery and psychospiritual transformation. For these reasons, maternal educators need to be educated in spirituality and be flexible, integrative and open in the spiritual shared journey of discovery. The point of this maternal education is to create and foster wholeness. When 'intuition couples with intellect, and the passions of the heart unite with those of the mind, then transformative knowledge is gained' (Root-Bernstein and Root-Bernstein 1999, 325).

The importance of spirituality in the birthing woman, and in diverse crises and traumas that may befall the mother through her life, is established in the research. The literature shows that implementing support, education and care for both the mother and the caregiver is paramount going forward in their spiritual and mental wellbeing.

Conclusions

It is important to note that this study was limited in its population sample to biological mothers, i.e. all participants were the biological mothers of their children, therefore, their desire for reproduction was conceptualised in the experience of the 'embodied knowing'. However, motherhood is changing in contemporary times. Many mothers are assisted by reproductive technology. Results in this study cannot be generalised to all mothers in the future, as they were all biological mothers. Research needs to be done on women who do not go through pregnancy or birth, yet are still mothers, and whether they are affected by embodied spirituality.

The study was limited in its population sample to ethnically white women. In previous research, it has been evident that the experience of motherhood is affected by the interaction of ethnicity and gender. Minority ethnic groups in the West, such as black women and/or Asian women, may experience various forms of oppression simultaneously (Craddock 2015; Griffith 2010; Radey and Brewster 2007; Sangha and Gonsalves 2013). Thus, the results in this study cannot be applied to all mothers, as the study concentrates on 'white motherhood', and the cultural, social and economic realities of that particular ethnicity.

Mothers in this study were middle-class women. The interaction between socio-economic background and the experience of motherhood is very complex. Results in this study, therefore, cannot be applied to lower-income mothers and their maternal experiences. All mothers were married/heterosexual women, a status which is also significant in motherhood experiences. Single motherhood, 'queer' motherhood and other arrangements will inevitably impact greatly on all aspects of the maternal experience, including spirituality. Therefore, this study opens many vistas for future research. Interdisciplinary pathways for researching spirituality issues related to motherhood have been identified, as well as the complex inter-actions of the maternal transition with those who help and assist in it.

In ancient societies, human beings used to live in a community and enjoy large family gatherings; the expectant mother was spiritually prepared for her role and the new mother was catered for and supported throughout pregnancy and later on in the postnatal period. While it is not about looking romantically or nostalgically at a pre-modern, spiritually-literate society (because that experience is not possible), in the Western world the postmodern, postindustrialised, postsecular and pluralised society, with mostly nuclear families, we face unique challenges in adopting or reinventing the notion of spiritual care. I believe, as a consequence of this study, that spiritual care needs to be adapted to the post-modern cultural milieu, including the technological revolution in which mothers' voices are very active.

It is paramount for mothers to develop internal structures. I believe these structures are needed to facilitate the intimate connection that mothers need to cultivate with themselves, and ultimately in their engagement with their children. My understanding is that this process/journey is about the capacity to develop a maternal, spiritual attunement. This maternal, spiritual attunement is the source from which to develop an internal conscious map. Spiritual skills/capacities can help at developing this conscious map by enabling mothers to access and connect parts of themselves, and also the environment, in relation to the adaptation and harmonious integration of their maternal experiences.

Note

1 For an introductory vision on integral studies and the future of integral theory, see: http://cejournal.org/GRD/Mapmaking.pdf.

References

Ayers-Gould, J. 2000. 'Spirituality in Birth: Creating Sacred Space within the Medical Model'. *International Journal of Childbirth Education* 15(1):14–17.

Baker, J. 1992. 'The Shamanic Dimensions of Childbirth'. *Pre- and Peri-natal Psychology Journal* 7(1):5–20.

Balin, J. 1988. 'The Sacred Dimensions of Pregnancy and Birth'. *Qualitative Sociology* 11(4):275–301.

Beck, D., and Cowan, C. 2005. *Spiral Dynamics: Mastering Values, Leadership and Change*. Victoria, Australia: Blackwell Publishing.

Budin, W. 2001. 'Birth and Death: Opportunities for Self-Transcendence'. *Journal Perinatal Education* 10(2):38–42.

Burns, E. 2015. 'The Blessingway Ceremony: Ritual, Nostalgic Imagination and Feminist Spirituality'. *Journal of Religious Health* 54(2):783–797.

Callister, L. 2010. 'Spirituality in Childbearing Women'. *Journal of Perinatal Education* 19(2):16–24.

Craddock, K. 2015. *Black Motherhood(s): Contexts, Contours and Considerations.* Ontario, Canada: Demeter Press.

Crowther, S. 2013. 'Sacred Space at the Moment of Birth'. *Practical Midwife* 16(11):21–23.

Crowther, S., and Hall, J. 2015. 'Spirituality and Spiritual Care in and around Childbirth'. *Women and Birth* 28(2):173–178.

Davies, S., and Coldridge, L. 2015. '"No Man's Land": An Exploration of the Traumatic Experiences of Student Midwives in Practice'. *Midwifery* 31(9):858–864.

Fisher, V., and Bickel, B. 2005. 'Awakening the Divine Feminine: A Stepmother-Daughter Collaborative Journey through Art-Making and Ritual in Mothering, Religion and Spirituality'. *Journal of the Association for Research on Mothering* 7(1):52–67.

Gebser, J. 1986. *The Ever-Present Origin: The Foundations and Manifestations of the Perspectival World.* Ohio, USA: Ohio University Press.

Graves, C. 1970. 'Levels of Existence: An Open System Theory of Values'. *Journal of Humanistic Psychology* 10(2):131–155.

Griffith, L. 2010. 'Motherhood, Ethnicity and Experience: A Narrative Analysis of the Debates Concerning Culture in the Provision of Health Services for Bangladeshi Mothers in East London'. *Anthropology and Medicine Journal* 17(3):289–299.

Heinz, A., Disney, E., Epstein, D., Glezen, L., Clark, P., and Preston, K. 2010. 'A Focus-Group Study on Spirituality and Substance-Abuse Treatment'. *Substance Use Misuse* 4(1–2):134–153.

Hitchcock, J., Schubert, P., and Thomas, S. 2003. *Community Health Nursing: Caring in Action.* Andover, UK: Cengage Learning.

Hover-Kramer, D. 2002. *Healing Touch: Guide Book for Practitioners.* Andover, UK: Cengage Learning.

Klassen, C. 2005. 'The Infertile Goddess: A Challenge to Maternal Imagery in Feminist Witchcraft in Mothering, Religion and Spirituality'. *Journal of the Association for Research on Mothering* 7(1):45–51.

Lahood, G. 2007. 'Rumour of Angels and Heavenly Midwives: Anthropology of Transpersonal Events and Childbirth'. *Women and Birth* 20(7):3–10.

Leinweber, J., and Rowe, H. 2010. 'The Costs of "Being with the Woman": Secondary Traumatic Stress in Midwifery'. *Midwifery* 26:76–87.

Mann, J. R., McKeown, R. E., Bacon, J., Vesselinov, R., and Bush, F. 2007. 'Religiosity, Spirituality, and Depressive Symptoms in Pregnant Women'. *International Journal of Psychiatry in Medicine* 37(3):301–313.

Mann, J. R., McKeown, R. E., Bacon, J., Vesselinov, R., and Bush, F. 2008. 'Do Antenatal Religious and Spiritual Factors Impact the Risk of Postpartum Depressive Symptoms?'. *Journal of Women's Health* 17(5):745–755.

Manning, L., and Radina, M. 2015. 'The Role of Spirituality in the Lives of Mothers of Breast Cancer Survivors'. *Journal of Religion, Spiritual and Aging* 1:27(2–3):125–144.

Moloney, S., and Gair, S. 2015. 'Empathy and Spiritual Care in Midwifery Practice: Contributing to Women's Enhanced Birth Experiences'. *Women Birth* 28(4):323–328.

Nuzum, D., Meaney, S., and O' Donoghue, K. 2014. 'The Provision of Spiritual and Pastoral Care following Stillbirth in Ireland: A Mixed Methods Study'. *BMJ Supportive Palliative Care*. [Epub ahead of print].

Nuzum, D., Meaney, S., O'Donoghue, K., and Morris, H. 2015. 'The Spiritual and Theological Issues Raised by Stillbirth for Healthcare Chaplains'. *Journal of Pastoral Care and Counselling* 69(3):163–170.

Radey, M., and Brewster, K. 2007. 'The Influence of Race/Ethnicity on Disadvantaged Mothers' Child Care Arrangements'. *Early Childhood Research Quarterly* 22:379–393.

Rice, H., and Warland, J. 2013. 'Bearing Witness: Midwives Experiences of Witnessing Traumatic Birth'. *Midwifery* 29(9):1056–1063.

Root-Bernstein, R., and Root-Bernstein, M. 1999. *Sparks of Genius: The Thirteen Thinking Tools of the World's Most Creative People.* New York: Houghton Mifflin.

Sangha, J., and Gonsalves, T. 2013. *South Asian Mothering – Negotiating Culture, Family and Selfhood.* Ontario, Canada: Demeter Press.

Sempruch, J. 2005. 'The Sacred Mothers, the Evil Witches and the Politics of Household in Toni Morrison's Paradise in Mothering, Religion and Spirituality'. *Journal of the Association for Research on Mothering* 7(1):98–109.

Sered, S. 1991. 'Childbirth as a Religious Experience? Voices from an Israeli Hospital'. *Journal of Feminist Studies in Religion* 7(2):7–18.

Snodgrass, J. 2012. 'A Psychospiritual, Family-Centered Theory of Care for Mothers in the NICU'. *Journal Pastoral Care Counsel* 66(1):2.

Wilber, K. 1986. *Transformations of Consciousness: Conventional and Contemplative Perspectives on Development.* Boston, USA: Shambhala New Science Library.

Wilber, K. 1997. *The Eye of Spirit: An Integral Vision for a World Gone Slightly Mad.* Boston, USA: Shambhala.

Wilber, K. 2007. *The Integral Vision: A Very Short Introduction to the Revolutionary Integral Approach to Life, God, the Universe, and Everything.* Boston, USA: Shambhala.

Woodhouse, M. 1996. *Paradigm Wars: Worldviews for a New Age.* Berkeley, USA: Frog Ltd.

Index

Page numbers in **bold** denote tables, those in *italics* denote figures.

Printed in the United States
by Baker & Taylor Publisher Services

Printed in the United States
by Baker & Taylor Publisher Services